CLINICAL COMPANION
to Accompany
MEDICAL-SURGICAL NURSING
An Integrated Approach, 2nd Edition

CLINICAL COMPANION
to Accompany
MEDICAL-SURGICAL NURSING
An Integrated Approach.
2nd Edition

Lois White, RN, PhD
Former Chairperson, Professor
Department of Vocational Nurse Education
Del Mar College
Corpus Christi, Texas

Gena Duncan, RN, MSN, MSEd
Assistant Professor and
Director of Associate Degree
Nursing Program
University of St. Francis
Fort Wayne, Indiana

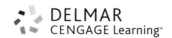

Australia • Brazil • Japan • Korea • Mexico • Singapore • Spain • United Kingdom • United States

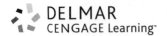
DELMAR
CENGAGE Learning™

Clinical Companion to Accompany
Medical-Surgical Nursing:
An Integrated Approach,
Second Edition
Lois White, Gena Duncan

Business Unit Director:
William Brottmiller

Executive Editor: Cathy L Esperti

Acquisitions Editor:
Matthew Filimonov

Senior Developmental Editor:
Elisabeth F. Williams

Editorial Assistant: Melissa Longo

Executive Marketing Manager:
Dawn F. Gerrain

Channel Manager: Tara Carter

Project Editor:
Maureen M. E. Grealish

Production Coordinator:
Anne Sherman

Senior Art/Design Coordinator:
Timothy J. Conners

For product information and technology assistance, contact us at
Cengage Learning Customer & Sales Support, 1-800-354-9706

For permission to use material from this text or product,
submit all requests online at **www.cengage.com/permissions**
Further permissions questions can be emailed to
permissionrequest@cengage.com

Library of Congress Control Number: 2001028702

ISBN-13: 978-0-7668-2567-3

ISBN-10: 0-7668-2567-1

Delmar
Executive Woods
5 Maxwell Drive
Clifton Park, NY 12065
USA

Cengage Learning is a leading provider of customized learning solutions
with office locations around the globe, including Singapore, the United
Kingdom, Australia, Mexico, Brazil, and Japan. Locate your local office at
international.cengage.com/region

Cengage Learning products are represented in Canada by
Nelson Education, Ltd.

To learn more about Delmar, visit **www.cengage.com/delmar**

Purchase any of our products at your local college store or at our
preferred online store **www.ichapters.com**

Notice to the Reader
Publisher does not warrant or guarantee any of the products described herein or perform any independent analysis in
connection with any of the product information contained herein. Publisher does not assume, and expressly disclaims, any
obligation to obtain and include information other than that provided to it by the manufacturer. The reader is expressly warned
to consider and adopt all safety precautions that might be indicated by the activities described herein and to avoid all potential
hazards. By following the instructions contained herein, the reader willingly assumes all risks in connection with such instructions. The publisher makes no representations or warranties of any kind, including but not limited to, the warranties of fitness
for particular purpose or merchantability, nor are any such representations implied with respect to the material set forth
herein, and the publisher takes no responsibility with respect to such material. The publisher shall not be liable for any special,
consequential, or exemplary damages resulting, in whole or part, from the readers' use of, or reliance upon, this material.

Printed in the United States of America
2 3 4 5 6 7 11 10 09

CONTENTS

PREFACE

Quality care of clients in the clinical area requires a vast amount of knowledge. Often a little reminder or quick reference assists the nurse in providing that quality care. Developed specifically for the Practical/Vocational nurse, this *Companion* is intended to be such a guide or quick-reference. Adapting only the most pertinent clinical information from *Medical-Surgical Nursing: An Integrated Approach,* 2nd edition, this volume is an invaluable tool for practicing and student nurses alike.

ORGANIZATION

The *Clinical Companion* follows the organization of the *Medical-Surgical Nursing, 2E.* It contains 37 chapters (the final chapter on critical thinking is not included) and is divided into 11 units. Each chapter highlights essential information from the corresponding chapter in the parent text.

The first 15 chapters provide factors and concepts basic to providing quality client care. The easy-to-read bulleted lists of the remaining chapters remind the user of assessments, diagnostic tests, and treatments generally used for the various body systems and/or disorders. The balance of the chapters focus on specific issues associated with providing client care.

FEATURES

- Easy-to-read bulleted lists of information significant to the clinical area.
- Charts contrasting similar diseases.
- General protocols for client care before, during, and following diagnostic tests.
- Quick reference for abbreviations.
- List of NANDA nursing diagnoses.

FOUNDATIONS OF NURSING

UNIT 1
Factors Affecting Nursing Care

UNIT 2
Holistic Nursing Care

THE HEALTH CARE DELIVERY SYSTEM

A health care delivery system is a mechanism for providing services that meet the health-related needs of individuals.

TYPES OF HEALTH CARE SERVICES

Health care services can be classified into three levels: primary, secondary, and tertiary. The trend is toward holistic care, that is, care of the entire person including physiological, psychological, social, intellectual, and spiritual aspects.

Primary Care

The major purposes of primary care are to promote wellness and prevent illness or disability.

Secondary Care

Services within the realm of secondary care—diagnosis and treatment—occur after the client exhibits symptoms of illness. Acute treatment centers (hospitals) constitute the predominant site for the delivery of these health care services.

Tertiary Care

Restoring an individual to the state of health that existed before the development of an illness is the purpose of tertiary (rehabilitative) care.

HEALTH CARE DELIVERY SYSTEM

The U.S. health care delivery system is complex, involving myriad providers, consumers, personnel, and services.

Providers/Consumers

Health care services in the United States are delivered by public (including official and voluntary), public/private, and private sectors. Consumers are the individuals who receive the health care services.

Public Sector

Public agencies are financed with tax monies; thus, these agencies are accountable to the public. The public sector includes official (or governmental) agencies and voluntary agencies.

Public/Private Sector

A blending of the public and private sectors in many areas of health care has gradually occurred following the inception of Medicare and the diagnosis-related groups (DRGs). Federal regulations guide both the care provided to clients in private non-profit and for-profit agencies by private physicians and the reimbursement to both the agencies and the physicians.

Private Sector

The private sector of the health care delivery system is composed primarily of independent health care agencies and providers who are reimbursed on a fee-for-service basis (the recipient directly pays the provider for services as they are provided). Fee-for-service clients may have private insurance or use their own financial resources to pay the provider for services rendered.

Personnel and Services

Many personnel and services exist within the various health care settings. Large hospitals provide the greatest number of services. Other health care settings may provide some but not all of these same services. The service departments most commonly found in the various settings include nursing units, specialized client care units, diagnostic departments, therapy departments, and support services.

Nursing Units

Nursing units are composed of client rooms, where most nursing care is provided. Units often serve one particular type of client such as cardiac, orthopedic, diabetic, surgical, pediatric, or obstetric. The nurse responsible for the unit may be called by several different titles, such as unit coordinator, nurse manager, or head nurse. Registered nurses (RNs), licensed practical/vocational nurses (LP/VNs), and nursing assistants provide the nursing care.

Specialized Client Care Units

Specialized units provide nursing care for specific needs of the clients. The LP/VN may work in these areas depending on experience, further education, the size and location of the hospital, and the number of RNs available. Examples of specialized units include the following:

- Emergency department (ED)
- Intensive care unit (ICU)
- Coronary care unit (CCU)
- Mental health unit
- Psychiatric unit
- Rehabilitation unit
- Dialysis unit
- Hospice unit
- Outpatient unit
- Home care
- Client education unit

Surgical Units

Care of the client just before, during, and after surgery is performed by the operating room (OR) and recovery room (RR) personnel. In addition to the main surgical unit, many hospitals also have a day surgery/ambulatory surgery unit. Clients come in a couple of hours before their scheduled surgeries and leave when recovered from the anesthesia. Total length of stay is shorter than 24 hours.

Diagnostic Departments

Diagnostic departments provide specialized tests that assist the physician in making a diagnosis for the client.

CLINICAL LABORATORY Clinical laboratory personnel examine specimens of tissues, feces, and body fluids such as blood, sputum, urine, amniotic fluid, and spinal fluid. Testing assesses values of normal components as well as abnormal components of these specimens.

RADIOLOGY DEPARTMENT X-ray studies are performed in the radiology department, sometimes called nuclear medicine. This department also performs computed tomography (CT) scans, mammography, ultrasound, arteriograms, venograms, echocardiograms, and magnetic resonance imaging (MRI).

OTHER DIAGNOSTIC SERVICES Other diagnostic services may include the following:

- Sleep center: provides observation, testing, and monitoring of clients as they sleep, to identify sleep-related problems
- Electroencephalography (EEG): records brain waves and ascertains electrical activity in the brain
- Electrocardiogram (ECG): records electrical activity in the heart
- Electromyogram (EMG): records electrical activity in body muscles

Therapy Departments

The function of the various therapy departments is to provide specialized treatments and/or rehabilitation services to clients to improve functional level in a specific area. Most hospitals have respiratory therapy and physical therapy departments. Some large teaching hospitals also have occupational therapy and speech therapy departments.

Support Services

Support services meet various other needs in providing care to clients.

- Pharmacists
- Dietitians
- Social workers
- Chaplains
- Admission department
- Business office
- Medical records
- Housekeeping and maintenance

HEALTH CARE TEAM

Health care services are delivered by a multidisciplinary team. Because nurses work with the other team members on an ongoing basis, it is necessary to understand the role of each team member.

Nurses function in independent, interdependent, and dependent roles. In the independent role, the nurse requires no direction or order from another health care professional, for example, in deciding that a client's edematous arm should be elevated. In the interdependent role, the nurse works in collaboration with other health care professionals, for example, in a client care conference where several members of the health care team together plan ways to meet the client's needs. In the dependent role, the nurse requires direction from a physician or dentist, for example, medications must be ordered by a physician or dentist before a nurse may administer them to the client. The degree of autonomy nurses experience is related to client needs, nurse expertise, and practice setting.

FACTORS INFLUENCING HEALTH CARE

Despite cost-containment efforts (such as DRGs, established by the federal government, and managed care, established by the insurers), the U.S. health care system still has problems with issues of cost, access, and quality. These issues are important for nurses to understand and are integral to any effort toward health reform.

CHALLENGES WITHIN THE HEALTH CARE SYSTEM

The major challenges facing the U.S. health care delivery system—which also happen to impact the control of costs—include the public's disillusionment with providers; providers' and consumers' loss of control over health care decisions; decreased use of hospitals and the accompanying negative impact on quality of care; changing practice settings; ethical issues; and vulnerable populations.

Ethical Issues

The United States is struggling with a major ethical conflict of cost containment versus compassionate care.

NURSING'S RESPONSE TO HEALTH CARE CHALLENGES

As the United States continues to look for ways to address the issue of health care reform, the implications for nursing will continue to increase. Some nurses feel threatened by impending changes, whereas others are excited about the possibility of transforming the health care system into something better.

Standards of Care

Another approach to the challenges of the health care delivery system has been the move toward standardization of care. There is significant variation in the diagnosis and treatment of certain illnesses and diseases. The Agency for Health Care Policy and Research (AHCPR) aims to identify the standards of treatment to which the health care community can be held. Currently, 18 AHCPR-published guidelines are available to the public and should be integral to nursing practice.

Public Health

During the past several years, public health has perceptibly eroded. Public health includes services such as immunizations, prenatal care, environmental concerns (conditions that may affect health), and analysis of the prevailing disease patterns in a community.

Community Health

Community-based care focuses on prevention and primary care. Successful movement toward a healthy and empowered consumer requires access to community-based primary health care.

SUGGESTED READING

Feldstein, P. J. (1999). *Health care economics* (5th ed.). Albany, NY: Delmar.

Hull, K. (1997). Hospital trends. In C. Harrington & C. L. Estes (Eds.), *Health policy and nursing: Crisis and reform in the U.S. health care delivery system* (2nd ed). Boston: Jones & Bartlett.

Kellogg Foundation. (1994). *How people view their providers. Report of a survey.* Battle Creek, MI: Author.

News. (2000). High public esteem for nurses. *AJN 100*(1), 21.

Zerwekh, J., & Claborn, J. C. (1997). *Nursing today: Transitions and trends.* Philadelphia: W. B. Saunders.

CRITICAL THINKING

Thinking as a nurse involves much more than gathering an assortment of facts and skills. Critical thinking in nursing education is an integral component of the curriculum.

Nurses in clinical practice are challenged to improve their ability to reason clearly and logically.

CRITICAL THINKING

The first step in improving the ability to think well is to develop an understanding of critical thinking. Each person must learn to be reflective, or introspective, about his or her own thinking. Quality thinking is like any skill; it takes practice and discipline to learn.

SKILLS OF CRITICAL THINKING

Four basic skills are necessary for the development of higher-level thinking skills. These skills are part of the process of developing and using thinking for problem-solving and reasoning. The four basic skills are critical reading, critical listening, critical writing, and critical speaking.

REASONING AND PROBLEM-SOLVING

Reasoning has been defined as the process of figuring things out by using critical thinking skills. Although reasoning involves thinking, all thinking is not reasoning. In order to use reasoning, to figure things out, or to problem-solve, the student must become familiar with the components of reasoning. These elements are purpose, the question at issue, assumptions, point of view, data and information, concepts, inferences and conclusions, and implications and consequences.

Professional Tip: Critical Thinking

Critical thinking is far more than an academic exercise. As a nurse, you are responsible for helping clients achieve and maintain their optimal level of health. To help sharpen your critical thinking skills, get in the habit of asking yourself several times throughout the day while caring for clients questions such as "Why is this procedure being done?", "What are its benefits?", and "Do I see alternatives that might result in better client outcomes?" Training yourself to think critically about all client care and interactions will help you to become a more skilled and compassionate professional.

LEGAL RESPONSIBILITIES

Nursing, which embodies a concern for the client in every aspect of life, encompasses a great responsibility—one that requires knowledge, skill, care, and commitment. As society advances and technology changes, the issues that affect nursing practice also change. We continue to recognize the importance of informed consent, the right to decide what is best for one's self, and belief in the client's bill of rights. However, difficult issues, such as living wills, advance directives, do-not-resuscitate (DNR) orders, and impaired nurses, now confront the profession of nursing. Nurses in the past did not have to contend with these controversial topics. Today's nurse must be informed on these and other issues.

All fifty states and the District of Columbia have enacted Good Samaritan laws which protect health care providers by ensuring immunity from civil liability (obligation one has incurred or might incur through any act or failure to act) when care is provided at the scene of an emergency and the caregiver does not intentionally or recklessly cause the client injury (Brown, 1999).

The Good Samaritan law applies only in emergency situations, usually those outside the hospital setting. It stipulates that the health care worker must not be acting for an employer or receive compensation for care given. There is also a federal Good Samaritan law that protects health care providers who voluntarily give care to a person in distress during an airplane flight (Brown, 1999).

NURSING PRACTICE AND THE LAW

In most states, nurses are bound by rules and regulations stipulated by the nursing practice act as determined by the legislature. For licensed practical/vocational nurses (LP/VNs) four states, Texas, California, Tennessee, and South Dakota, have title acts as opposed to practice acts. Nursing practice acts state those things that the nurse can and cannot do, whereas title acts state who can be called an LP/VN.

Under the auspices of the nursing practice acts, guidelines have been developed to direct nursing care. These guidelines are called standards of practice or standards of care. The nurse is expected to act in a reasonable and prudent manner.

Liability

What is meant by reasonable and prudent? In the case of nursing, it means that the nurse is expected to act as would other nurses at the same professional level and with the same amount of education or experience. If most nurses would respond to a particular situation in a certain way, and the nurse in question does so also, the nurse would be acting in a reasonable and prudent manner. Liability is determined by whether the nurse adhered to the standards of practice.

Legal Issues in Practice

Nurses are responsible for their actions regardless of who told them to perform those actions. A nurse who leaves an inadequately staffed unit could be charged with client abandonment.

NURSE-CLIENT RELATIONSHIP

A variety of situations can develop between a nurse and a client that may require legal intervention. The following is a discussion of the types of torts that may arise.

Intentional Torts

An intentional tort is a knowing or willful violation of another individual's civil rights.

Assault and Battery

Assault and battery, though frequently used together, are actually two separate terms. Assault is the threat to do something that may cause harm or be unpleasant to another person. Battery is the unauthorized or unwanted touching of one person by another.

Fear and intimidation are the key elements in assault. The person assaulted must believe that the threat made can and will be carried out.

The key factor regarding battery is consent. People have the right to be free of unwanted handling of their person. Striking a client is battery. Performing a procedure without the client's consent is battery. Forcing a person to take medication they do not want is battery. Any unwanted touching, regardless of outcome, can be construed as battery.

Defamation

Defamation is the use of words to harm or injure the personal or professional reputation of another person. If the words are written down, they constitute libel. If the information is communicated verbally to a third party, it constitutes slander.

The most common examples of this tort are giving out inaccurate or inappropriate information from the medical record; discussing clients, families, or visitors in public areas; or speaking negatively about coworkers (Zerwekh & Claborn, 1997).

Fraud

Fraud is a wrong that results from a deliberate deception intended to produce unlawful gain. Common forms of fraud in health care include illegal billing and deceit in obtaining or attempting to obtain a nursing license (Flight, 1998).

False Imprisonment

False imprisonment refers to making the client wrongfully believe that she cannot leave a place. The most common example of this tort is telling a client not to leave the hospital until the bill is paid (Zerwekh & Claborn, 1997). Any mechanism used to confine a client or to restrict movement can be considered a restraint and a form of false imprisonment. This includes threats, locked doors, physical restraints such as wrist or vest restraints, side rails, geriatric chairs, and psychotropic drugs.

The client in restraints must be assessed frequently. Documentation must show that:

- Restraints were checked hourly and released every 2 hours,
- The client was toileted,
- The client received food and water, and
- The client had position changes.

In acute care settings, restraints can usually be applied temporarily as a nursing measure for client safety; however, in most states, a physician's order must be immediately obtained. In long-term care settings, a physician's order is required prior to utilizing any restraints.

Invasion of Privacy

Privacy includes the right to be left alone, to choose care based on personal beliefs, to govern body integrity, and to choose when and how sensitive information is shared (Badzek & Gross, 1999). People are entitled to confidential (nondisclosure of information) treatment regarding health care. All information gleaned from working with a client or his medical records must be kept confidential. Therefore, a client's health status may not be discussed with a third party, unless either the client is present and has given verbal permission or permission has been obtained in writing. This does not apply to nurses' discussing a client's health status with other health care workers involved in the care of the client.

A common mistake made by health care personnel is discussing clients in public areas. It is difficult to gauge who may overhear when comments are made while sitting in the cafeteria or waiting for the elevator.

Unintentional Torts

Negligence and malpractice are considered to be unintentional torts.

Negligence

Negligence is a general term referring to negligent or careless acts on the part of an individual who is not exercising reasonable or prudent judgment.

Malpractice

Negligent acts on the part of a professional can be termed malpractice, or professional negligence. More specifically, malpractice relates to the conduct of a person while acting in a professional capacity. Negligent or careless acts on the part of a nurse frequently come from not meeting the standards of care, in other words, from not doing what a reasonable and prudent nurse would do under similar circumstances. A nurse can be charged with malpractice for acts committed or acts omitted.

The prudent nurse is protected by adhering to facility policy and procedure and attempting to meet the standards of care at all times.

Documentation

The source of information regarding the client's clinical history is the medical record, or the chart. The chart should accurately reflect diagnosis, treatment, testing, clinical course, nursing assessment, and intervention. According to the law, "If it was not charted, it was not done." If a chart ever winds up in court, this is the standard the jury applies when trying to determine what happened and who is at fault.

The nurse should not chart medications before they are given or treatments before they are completed. All client care, including treatments, is documented *after* being provided.

Documentation must be accurate and objective; that is, it should reflect facts, not inferences or opinions, about the client.

Entries must be neat, legible, spelled correctly, written clearly, and signed or initialed. It is illegal to go back and change a chart. If an error in charting is made, a line should be drawn through the incorrect entry and the nurse should initial it. Blacking out entries or using correction fluid is not acceptable, as this renders the original entry illegible. Sloppy, misspelled charting might discredit excellent nursing care.

INFORMED CONSENT

Informed consent refers to a competent client's ability to make health care decisions based on full disclosure of the benefits, risks, potential

consequences of a recommended treatment plan, and alternate treatments, including no treatment and the client's agreement to the treatment as indicated by the client's signing a consent form. This detailed explanation, provided by the physician, allows the client to make intelligent decisions about treatment options. The issue of informed consent deals with the right of the client to determine what happens to his or her person. Consent to treatment also helps protect the health care worker from unwarranted charges of battery. Consent may be withdrawn, either verbally or in writing, at any time.

Individuals who are declared incompetent have a guardian or someone who has power of attorney to make heath care decisions and give consent for treatment.

Nurses must obtain consent for nursing procedures. Each client, on admission, signs a general care consent form. The nurse is obligated to explain what is to be done to the client and to receive at least implied consent, as indicated by lack of objection on the part of the client. It is the physician's responsibility to obtain consent for medical or surgical treatment. Student nurses should neither ask the client to sign a consent form, nor witness a consent form.

Invasive procedures or those that may have serious consequences, such as surgery, cardiac catheterization, or HIV testing, require written consent. Consent for procedures that are not invasive can be either given verbally or implied. Consent is implied when immediate action is necessary to save a life or prevent permanent physical harm. Written consent is waived. After the emergency is over, consent must be obtained for further care.

ADVANCE DIRECTIVES

An advance directive is a written instruction for health care that is recognized under state law and is related to the provision of such care when the individual is incapacitated. Advance directives emphasize the right of the client to self-determination. They are instructions about health care preferences regarding life-sustaining measures. When an advance directive indicates that the client does not wish to have cardiopulmonary resuscitation (CPR) performed in the event of cardiac arrest, the physician must write a DNR order, also referred to as a "No Code."

All health care facilities that receive Medicare or Medicaid monies are required to offer to all competent clients on admission the opportunity to execute advance directives. The medical record must show that the client was offered the opportunity to complete these documents. The documentation must indicate decisions made or not made at that time. Clients cannot be coerced into signing advance directives, nor can they be discriminated against should they choose not to sign an advance directive.

Durable Power of Attorney

A durable power of attorney for health care (DPAHC) is a legal document designating who may make health care decisions for a client when that client is no longer capable of decision making. This health care representative is appointed by the client and is expected to act in the best interests of the client. This appointment can be revoked any time the competent client chooses.

Living Will

A living will is a legal document that allows a person to state preferences about the use of life-sustaining measures should she be unable to make her wishes known.

INCIDENT REPORTS

An incident report is a risk management tool used to describe and report any unusual event that occurs to a client, visitor, or staff member. Incident reports are completed to document such events as falls, medication errors, forgotten treatment, injuries—anything that happens out of the ordinary. Another name for an incident report is a variance report or an occurrence report.

IMPAIRED NURSE

By definition, an impaired nurse is a nurse who is habitually intemperate or is addicted to the use of alcohol or habit-forming drugs. In many states, the board of nursing requires nurses to report impaired coworkers. Nurses suspected of being under the influence of drugs or alcohol must be reported to the proper authority at the place of employment. The second consideration is getting help for the impaired nurse and taking action to correct the problem.

A nurse who suspects a coworker of diverting drugs or abusing alcohol should:

1. Document the dates, times, and observed behavior. Specific and descriptive accounts of what was observed are critical. For example:

   January 3, 2000. P.P. working 3–11 shift. Client A and Client B verbalized unrelieved post-operative pain. Documentation by P.P. stated both clients were comfortable after administration of Demerol 75 mg IM. Narcotic count at shift change satisfactory.

   January 4, 2000. Client C and Client D verbalized unrelieved pain. Documentation by P.P. indicated both clients stated pain was relieved after administration of Demerol 100 mg IM. Narcotic count at shift change okay.

   January 5, 2000. Narcotic count showed 1 Demerol 100-mg syringe listed as broken and 1 Demerol 75-mg syringe listed as wasted, "client changed her mind." P.P. signed the narcotic sheet.

   March 1–2, 2000. S.L. working the night shift. Strong odor of alcohol on his breath.

   March 3, 2000. S.L. observed walking with unsteady gait, speech is slurred, strong odor of alcohol on breath.

2. Go to the supervisor and report concerns. Providing a copy of the documentation about the suspicious incidents is helpful.
3. Refrain from approaching or confronting the coworker.

REFERENCES

Badzek, L., & Gross, L. (1999). Confidentiality and privacy: At the forefront for nurses. *AJN, 99*(6), 52–54.

Brown, S. (1999). Good Samaritan laws: Protection and limits. *RN, 62*(11), 65.

Flight, M. (1998). *Law, liability, and ethics* (3rd ed.). Albany, NY: Delmar.

Zerwekh, J., & Claborn, J. C. (1997). *Nursing today: Transitions and trends.* (2nd ed.). Philadelphia: W. B. Saunders.

ETHICAL RESPONSIBILITIES

4

The delivery of ethical health care is becoming an increasingly difficult and confusing issue in contemporary society. Nurses are committed to respecting their clients' rights in terms of providing health care and treatment. This desire to maintain clients' rights, however, often conflicts with professional duties and institutional policies. Nurses must thus learn to balance these potentially conflicting perspectives so as to achieve the primary objective—the care of the client.

CONCEPT OF ETHICS

Ethics deals with one's responsibilities (duties and obligations) as defined by logical argument. Ethics looks at human behavior—which things people do under which types of circumstances. But ethics is not merely philosophical in nature; ethical persons put their beliefs into action.

Ethics in Health Care

The application of general ethical principles to health care is referred to as bioethics. Ethics affects every area of health care, including direct care of clients, allocation of finances, and utilization of staff. Ethics does not provide easy answers, but it can help provide structure by raising questions that ultimately lead to answers.

Every day, nurses face situations wherein they must make decisions that transcend technical and professional concerns. These situations may or may not be life threatening. Such situations raise complex problems that cannot be answered completely with technical knowledge and professional expertise. The way that nurses relate to clients, families, and other health care providers is the true demonstration of ethical behavior.

ETHICAL PRINCIPLES

Ethical principles are codes that direct or govern actions. They are widely accepted and generally based on the humane aspects of society. Ethical decisions are principled, that is, they reflect what is best for the client and society.

By applying ethical principles, the nurse can become more systematic in solving ethical conflicts. Ethical principles can be used as guidelines in analyzing dilemmas; they can also serve as justification (rationale) for the resolution of ethical problems.

Autonomy

The principle of autonomy refers to the individual's right to choose and the individual's ability to act on that choice.

Competent clients have a right to self-determination, even if their decisions may result in self-harm. Probably one of the most difficult things for nurses to accept is that clients are ultimately responsible for themselves; they will do what they want to do.

Nonmaleficence

Nonmaleficence is the obligation to cause no harm to others. Harm can take many forms: physiological, psychological, social, financial, and/or spiritual. Nonmaleficence refers to both intentional harm and the risk of harm.

Beneficence

Beneficence is the duty to promote good and to prevent harm. Beneficence is often viewed as the core of nursing practice. The nurse serves as a client advocate and promotes the rights of the client. The nurse nurtures the client and incorporates the desires of the client into the plan of care.

Justice

The principle of justice is based on the concept of fairness extended to each individual. The major health-related issues of justice involve the way people are treated and the way resources are distributed.

Veracity

Veracity means truthfulness (neither lying nor deceiving others). Deception can take many forms: intentional lying, nondisclosure of information, or partial disclosure of information. Veracity often is difficult to achieve. It may not be hard to tell the truth, but it can be very hard to decide how much truth to tell. Exceptions to truth-telling are sometimes upheld by the principle of nonmaleficence, when the truth does greater harm than good. The act of giving placebo medications is an example of when telling the truth does greater harm than good.

Fidelity

The concept of fidelity (which is the ethical foundation of nurse–client relationships) means faithfulness and keeping promises.

Clients have an ethical right to expect nurses to act in their best interests. As nurses function in the role of client advocate (a person who speaks up for or acts on behalf of the client), they are upholding the principle of fidelity. Fidelity is demonstrated when nurses:

- Represent the client's viewpoint to other members of the health care team,
- Avoid letting their own personal values influence their advocacy for clients, and

• Support the client's decision, even when it conflicts with their own preferences or choices.

Within the nurse–client relationship, nurses should be loyal to their responsibilities, keep promises, maintain privacy, and meet resonable expectations of clients. Nurses also have a duty to be faithful to themselves.

ETHICAL CODES

One hallmark of a profession is the determination of ethical behavior for its members. The Code for Licensed Practical/Vocational Nurses, developed by the National Federation of Licensed Practical Nurses (NFLPN), is presented in Table 4–1. This code, adopted by NFLPN in 1961 and revised in 1979 and in 1991, provides a motivation for establishing, maintaining, and elevating professional standards. Each LP/VN, upon entering the profession, inherits the responsibility to adhere to the standards of ethical practice and conduct as set forth in this code.

THE CLIENT'S RIGHTS

Clients have certain rights that apply regardless of the setting for delivery of care. These rights include, but are not limited to, the right to:

• Make decisions regarding their care,
• Be actively involved in the treatment process, and
• Be treated with dignity and respect.

Table 4–1 THE CODE FOR LICENSED PRACTICAL/VOCATIONAL NURSES

1. Know the scope of maximum utilization of the LP/VN as specified by the nursing practice act and function within this scope.
2. Safeguard the confidential information acquired from any source about the patient.
3. Provide health care to all patients regardless of race, creed, cultural background, disease, or lifestyle.
4. Refuse to give endorsement to the sale and promotion of commercial products or services.
5. Uphold the highest standards in personal appearance, language, dress, and demeanor.
6. Stay informed about issues affecting the practice of nursing and delivery of health care and, where appropriate, participate in government and policy decisions.
7. Accept the responsibility for safe nursing by keeping oneself mentally and physically fit and educationally prepared to practice.
8. Accept responsibility for membership in NFLPN and participate in its efforts to maintain the established standards of nursing practice and employment policies which lead to quality patient care.

From Nursing Practice Standards for the Licensed Practical/Vocational Nurse, *by National Federation of Licensed Practical Nurses, Inc. (NFLPN), 1996, Garner, NC: Author. Copyright 1996 by Author. Reprinted with permission.*

ETHICAL DILEMMAS

An ethical dilemma occurs when there is a conflict between two or more ethical principles—when there is no "correct" decision. Ethical dilemmas are situations of conflicting requirements; something ought to be done and ought not to be done at the same time. Three areas where ethical dilemmas are possible are euthanasia, refusal of treatment, and scarcity of resources.

Euthanasia

In current times, euthanasia refers to intentional action or lack of action that causes the merciful death of someone suffering from a terminal illness or incurable condition.

Active euthanasia refers to taking deliberate action that will hasten the client's death, such as removing from a respirator a client who is in a vegetative state. In contrast, passive euthanasia means cooperating with the client's dying process. An example is not putting in a feeding tube to provide nourishment when the client cannot or will no longer eat.

Assisted suicide is a form of active euthanasia whereby another person provides a client with the means to end his own life. Regardless of a nurse's personal viewpoint, assisted suicide is still illegal.

Refusal of Treatment

The client's right to refuse treatment is based on the principle of autonomy. In fairness, the client can refuse treatment only after the treatment methods and their consequences have been explained. A client's rights to refuse treatment and to die challenge the values of most health care providers.

Scarcity of Resources

With the current emphasis on containing health care costs, the use of expensive services is being closely examined. The use of specialists, organ transplants, and distribution of services are being influenced by social and political forces.

In many situations, clients wait extended periods before receiving donated organs. The allocation of scarce resources is emerging as a major ethical dilemma.

ETHICAL DECISION MAKING

Nurses must understand the basis on which they make their decisions. Ethical reasoning is the process of thinking through what one ought to do in an orderly, systematic manner based on principles. Ethical decisions cannot be made in a scattered, unorganized manner based entirely on intuition or emotions. Ethical decision making is a rational way of making decisions in nursing practice. It is used in situations where either the right decision is not clear or conflicts of rights and duties exist.

Framework for Ethical Decision Making

When making an ethical decision, the nurse must consider the following relevant questions:

- Which theories are involved?
- Which principles are involved?

- Who will be affected?
- What will be the consequences of the alternatives (ethical options)?

The first step of ethical analysis is to gather relevant data in order to identify the ethical problem and to determine which type of ethical problem exists.

Next, all the people involved (the parties) must be considered. What are their rights, responsibilities, duties, and decision-making abilities? Who is the most appropriate person to make the decision? Whose problem is it? It is important to identify several possible alternatives and predict the outcome of each. Then, and only then, can a course of action be selected—one that, it is hoped, ends in resolution of the problem. The final step of ethical decision making is evaluation of the resolution process.

ETHICS AND NURSING

As professionals, nurses are accountable for protecting the rights and interests of the client. Whatever the setting, nurses must balance their ethical responsibilities to each client as an individual with their professional obligations. Often, there is an inherent conflict.

Ethics Committees

Many health care agencies now recognize the need for a systematic manner whereby to discuss ethical concerns. Ethics committees can lead to the establishment of policies and procedures for prevention and resolution of dilemmas.

Nurse as Client Advocate

When acting as a client advocate, the nurse's first step is to develop a meaningful relationship with the client. The nurse is then able to make decisions with the client based on the strength of the relationship. The nurse's primary ethical responsibility is to protect clients' rights to make their own decisions.

Nurse as Whistleblower

The term whistleblowing refers to calling public attention to unethical, illegal, or incompetent actions of others. Whistleblowing is based on the ethical principles of veracity and nonmaleficence. As professionals, nurses are expected to monitor coworkers' abilities to perform their duties safely.

Federal law and state laws (to varying degrees) provide protection, such as privacy, to whistleblowers. Unfortunately, however, the inclination to protect one's coworkers and the fear of reprisal may deter a nurse from fulfilling the ethical obligation to report substandard behaviors.

SUGGESTED READING

Haddad, A. (1999). Ethics in action. *RN, 62*(1), 23–26.

Schildmeier, D. (1997). Using public opinion to protect nursing practice. *AJN, 97*(3), 56–58.

Wolfe, S. (1999). Ethics on the job: A survey, quality vs. cost. *RN, 62*(1), 28–33.

COMMUNICATION

5

When communicating with a client, family, or another member of the health care team, it is important that the message be sent and received accurately.

METHODS OF COMMUNICATING

There are two methods of communicating: verbally and nonverbally.

Verbal Communication

Verbal communication is the use of words, either spoken or written, to send a message. Methods of verbal communication include speaking, listening, writing, and reading.

Speaking/Listening

Most commonly, speaking is thought of as verbal communication. The receiver of a spoken message must listen. Speaking and listening must both occur in order for there to be communication.

Writing/Reading

The other mode of verbal communication is writing. The receiver of the written message must read the words. The reader must understand the words and attach meaning to them. With a written message, immediate feedback is generally not available. Therefore, great care should be taken to ensure clarity when composing a written message.

Nonverbal Communication

Nonverbal communication, sometimes called body language, is the sending of a message without using words. There are many ways we communicate without words, including gestures, facial expressions, posture and gait, tone of voice, touch, eye contact, body position, and physical appearance.

Nonverbal communication is generally unconscious—part learned behavior and part instinct. Because there is little conscious control involved in nonverbal communication, feelings are generally most honestly expressed nonverbally.

Clients seem to believe and are particularly sensitive to nonverbal messages. Nurses must thus make an effort to be aware of the nonverbal messages they may be sending to clients.

Nurses must also be sensitive to the client's nonverbal messages. Many clients do not want to bother "busy" nurses. Such clients may say they are fine or do not need anything when this is in fact not the case.

INFLUENCES ON COMMUNICATION

Communication involves more than just the sending and receiving of verbal and nonverbal messages. How a person sends or receives a message is influenced by such factors as age, education, emotions, culture, and language.

CONGRUENCY OF MESSAGES

It is important that verbal and non-verbal communications be congruent, or in agreement. Incongruent messages can confuse the receiver, who then may require feedback in order to correctly interpret the message.

It is important for the nurse to watch for congruency between verbal and nonverbal messages and to ask for clarification when incongruity exists.

LISTENING/OBSERVING

Listening and observing are two of the most valuable skills a nurse can have.

The term active listening has been used to describe this behavior of listening and observing. The nurse who is at eye level with the client, who leans slightly forward toward the client, and who makes eye contact is showing undivided attention to the client and will be able to listen and

observe more accurately. Responses from the nurse such as "go on," "tell me more," "yes," "what else?" or "mmhm" both encourage the client to continue and communicate that the nurse is really listening.

THERAPEUTIC COMMUNICATION

Therapeutic communication, sometimes called effective communication, is purposeful and goal directed, creating a beneficial outcome for the client. One person is the helper (nurse) and the other is being helped (client). The focus of the conversation is the client, the client's needs, or the client's problems, not the needs or problems of the nurse.

Goals of Therapeutic Communication

One or more of these goals guide every therapeutic communication in the nurse–client relationship. The goals are: obtain or provide information, develop trust, show caring, and explore feelings.

Behaviors/Attitudes to Enhance Communication

Some behaviors and attitudes enhance therapeutic communication. Included are: self-disclosure, caring, genuineness, warmth, active listening, empathy, and acceptance and respect.

Techniques of Therapeutic Communication

Certain techniques promote therapeutic communication. These techniques should be learned and

Table 5–1   WAYS TO SHOW CARING

ACTIVITY	STATEMENTS TO USE WITH ACTIVITY
Cover the client with a blanket.	"It feels chilly in here. Perhaps this blanket will help."
Assist the client to dress.	"I noticed you're having a little trouble getting your robe on. Perhaps I can help."
Serve a tray to the client.	"It's time to eat. I hope you're hungry because it really looks good."
Offer assistance.	"Here, let me help you. Perhaps together we can arrange these flowers."
When leaving the room.	"Is there anything more I can do for you before I go?" or "I'm leaving now, but I'll be back in 20 minutes."
Move the client up in bed.	"You look so uncomfortable. Let me move you up in bed."
Make the client's bed.	"Now you have a nice fresh bed."
Regulate environmental temperature.	"It seems very warm in here. Perhaps if I turn the air conditioner up, it will help."
Turn the client in bed.	"Changing position really makes a difference, doesn't it?"
Straighten a pillow.	"Let me straighten your pillow for you."

Adapted from Mental Health Concepts *(4th ed.), by C. Waughfield, 1998, Albany, NY: Delmar. Copyright 1998 by Delmar. Adapted with permission.*

incorporated into the nurse's manner of communicating. The techniques are:

- Clarifying/validating
- Open questions
- Indirect statements
- Reflecting
- Paraphrasing
- Summarizing
- Focusing
- Silence

Barriers to Communication

The most common barriers are the following:

- Closed questions
- Clichés
- False reassurance
- Judgmental responses
- Agreeing/disagreeing or approving/disapproving
- Giving advice
- Stereotyping
- Belittling
- Defending
- Requesting an explanation
- Changing the subject

PSYCHOSOCIAL ASPECTS OF COMMUNICATION

The psychosocial aspects of communication include: style, gestures, meaning of time, meaning of space, cultural values, and political correctness. These aspects are based on individuality and culture and will influence the nurse–client relationship. It is important to understand these aspects and how they vary in different persons and cultures.

Effective communication has a positive influence on a client's well-being. Furthermore, clients often judge nurses' competence by their communication skills. Good communication skills also result in increased client satisfaction, and increased client satisfaction leads to increased compliance with the therapeutic regimen.

Communication, then, is a key factor in the client's perception and evaluation of the health care services provided.

NURSE–CLIENT COMMUNICATION

Factors Affecting Nurse–Client Communication

Factors affecting nurse–client communication include:

- Social factors
- Religion
- Family situation
- Visual ability—When caring for a patient who is visually impaired:
  —Look directly at the client when speaking.
  —Use a normal tone and volume of voice.
  —Advise the client when you are entering or leaving the room.
  —Orient the person to the immediate environment; use clock hours to indicate positions of items in relation to the client.
  —Ask for permission before touching the client.
- Hearing ability—Many persons

who are hearing impaired have learned, at least to some degree, to speechread, formerly known as lipread. Communicating with a client who is hearing impaired requires time and patience. The nurse should face the client and speak slowly and deliberately using slightly exaggerated word formation. Gesturing can also be very effective. Check to see whether the client has a hearing aid and, if so, encourage its use during the communication.
- Speech ability
- Level of consciousness—True communication cannot be accomplished with unconscious or comatose clients. It should be remembered, however, that unconscious or comatose clients can hear even though they cannot respond. Caregivers should speak to these clients just as they would to alert clients. Always greet the client by name, identify yourself, and explain why you are in the room (i.e., what you are going to do). Then let the client know when you are leaving and, if possible, when you will return. Although one-sided, this interaction is important to the client.
- Language proficiency—If another language is prevalent in the community, the nurse should learn some phrases in the language that are useful in client assessment and in care. Pictures or a two-language dictionary are often helpful. Remember, gestures and other nonverbal communication send messages without the use of language.
- Stage of illness

COMMUNICATING WITH THE HEALTH CARE TEAM

Oral communication among the health care team is necessary for the appropriate planned care of the client and for the efficient and effective functioning of the nursing unit. In order to provide continuity of care, all persons who provide direct care to clients must communicate orally with each other concerning that care.

Client care conferences may be scheduled regularly or whenever the need arises. Some conferences may be solely for the staff of a particular nursing unit; others may include members of other departments. In either case, only those persons directly involved with the care of the client should be invited.

Most written communication relates to the client's chart. All aspects of a client's care are recorded on that client's chart.

In many places, computers are used by client care departments to send requisitions to other departments and to receive test results.

COMMUNICATING WITH YOURSELF

Such communication often takes the form of thoughts rather than spoken words. What people say to themselves influences their personalities and, therefore, how they interact with others. Practicing positive self-talk is the key to positive self-esteem. Send positive thoughts to yourself about yourself. Remind yourself of your good attributes and accomplishments. Positive self-talk reinforces the desire to succeed.

Negative self-talk may originate within you, or you may be replaying things that others have said about you. Negative self-talk is self-destructive. Your self-image is lowered by your own criticism, and you begin to see yourself as a failure.

CULTURAL DIVERSITY AND NURSING

Every aspect of one's life—including attitudes, beliefs, and values—is influenced by one's culture. Behavior, including behavior affecting health, is culturally determined. As the population of the United States continues to diversify, recognition of cultural differences and their impact on health care becomes more critical. Nurses provide health care to culturally diverse client populations in a variety of settings. Knowledge of culturally relevant information is thus essential for delivery of competent nursing care.

CULTURE

To provide holistic care, the nurse needs a thorough understanding of concepts relating to culture. In society, culture refers to dynamic and integrated structures of knowledge, beliefs, behaviors, ideas, attitudes, values, habits, customs, languages, symbols, rituals, ceremonies, and practices that are unique to a particular group of people. This structure provides the group of people with a general design for living.

Culture is not static nor is it uniform among all members within a given cultural group. Culture represents adaptive dynamic processes learned through life experiences. Diversity among and within cultural groups results from individual perspectives and practices.

Ethnicity and Race

Ethnicity is a cultural group's perception of itself, or a group identity. Ethnicity is a sense of belongingness and a common social heritage that is passed from one generation to the next. Members of an ethnic group demonstrate their shared sense of identity through common customs and traits.

Race refers to a grouping of people based on biological similarities. Members of a racial group have similar physical characteristics such as blood group, facial features, and color of skin, hair, and eyes.

Cultural Diversity

Cultural diversity refers to the differences among people that result from racial, ethnic, and cultural variables. A variety of rich cultural heritages exist within the United States.

There are some disadvantages associated with living and working in such a culturally diverse society. Problems arise when differences across and within cultural groups are misunderstood. Misperception, confusion, and ignorance often accompany people's expectations of others.

Stereotyping is the belief that all people within the same racial, ethnic, or cultural group will act alike and share the same beliefs and attitudes. Stereotyping results in labeling people according to cultural preconceptions, thereby ignoring individual identity.

Characteristics of Culture

Five characteristics shared by all cultures are:

• Culture is learned.
• Culture is not inherited or innate, but, rather, culture is integrated throughout all the interrelated components.
• Culture is shared by everyone who belongs to the cultural group.
• Culture is tacit (unspoken), in that acceptable behavior is understood by everyone in the cultural group, regardless of whether beliefs are written down or spoken.
• Culture is dynamic; it is constantly changing.

CULTURAL INFLUENCES ON HEALTH CARE BELIEFS AND PRACTICES

It is common for cultural groups to have a body of knowledge and beliefs about health and disease. Cultural practices can positively and negatively affect health and disease distribution. Clients tend to define wellness and illness in the context of their own culture (Estin, 1999).

Beliefs of Select Cultural Groups

While the population of the United States encompasses innumerable ethnic groups, the European Americans, African Americans, Hispanic Americans, Asian Americans, and Native Americans together represent a majority.

European American

This ethnic group traces its origins to the Caucasian Protestants who came to this country from Northern Europe over 200 years ago. Values that still dominate the Caucasian American middle-class ethic include independence, individuality, wealth, comfort, cleanliness, achievement, punctuality, hard work, aggression, assertiveness, rationality, orientation toward the future, and mastery of one's own fate.

African American

African American ancestors came to North America from various African countries and the Caribbean as either slaves or free immigrants. The different countries of origin as well as disparate educational levels, income, occupations, and religious beliefs explain the heterogeneous (different) cultural practices among African Americans today.

Hispanic American

Although the Spanish language is common to most Hispanics, cultural patterns vary due to the different countries of origin. In general, the

Hispanic American belongs to a large extended-family system within which females are seen as subservient to males but as having a major role in family cohesiveness.

The influence of religion on culture is particularly evident in Hispanic populations. Western medicine is appropriate for some diseases, whereas the native healer (curandera) may have to intervene for illnesses having supernatural causes.

Asian American

Asian cultures are typically patrilineal, that is, family relations are traced through males. Males are the heads of household, and decision-makers, and elders are respected. Only physical complaints are acceptable, and maintaining eye contact is considered disrespectful (Estin, 1999).

Asians hold to a yin (cold) and yang (hot) etiology of disease. Illness occurs as a consequence of an imbalance in these forces. Many Asian Americans rely on herbal remedies, acupuncture, and cupping and burning, a treatment that draws blood to the skin's surface when a warmed cup is placed on the skin.

Native American

These peoples form a very diverse group, stemming from over 200 different tribes across the United States. Health is believed to result from a harmonious relationship with nature and the universe. Illness is frequently traced to a supernatural origin and discord with the forces of nature. Prevention may be attained through prayer, charms, and fetishes (objects having power to protect or aid the owner). Through prayers, rituals, ceremonies, and herbal drinks, health may be restored.

CULTURAL AND RACIAL INFLUENCES ON CLIENT CARE

In an unfamiliar situation, such as admission to a health care setting, cultural differences may seem even greater, because in times of stress, most people hold tightly to that which is familiar in order to protect themselves from the unknown. The nurse can show caring in such a situation by acknowledging the expression of these differences and encouraging the client to retain what is familiar.

The influences of culture and race can be viewed through the phenomena of communication, space and time orientation, social organization, and biological variations.

CULTURAL ASPECTS AND THE NURSING PROCESS

Nurses must be able to recognize the way that culture affects the health care needs of clients and respond appropriately.

Assessment

Culturally sensitive nursing care begins with an examination of one's own culture and beliefs. It is followed by an assessment of the client's cultural beliefs and background.

Client Cultural Assessment

There are six categories of information necessary for a comprehensive cultural assessment of the client:

- Ethnic or racial background
- Language and communication patterns
- Cultural values and norms
- Biocultural factors
- Religious beliefs and practices
- Health beliefs and practices

Nursing Diagnosis

Any nursing diagnosis may be appropriate for a client of any cultural group. When cultural variables are identified during assessment, the nurse should be as specific as possible when asking questions and determining appropriate nursing diagnoses, so that interventions can be individualized with respect to the client's cultural beliefs.

Planning/Outcome Identification

Cultural variables must be taken into consideration when establishing goals and planning interventions. Care will be most effective when the client and family are active participants in planning care, and when cultural preferences are respected.

Implementation

Cultural aspects are always a factor in a nursing care plan, and effective communication and client education are important nursing responsibilities that can enhance cultural understanding and appreciation. Interventions should be carried out in a manner that will respect, to the degree possible, the preferences and desires of the client. When a client does not speak or understand the native language well, the nurse should arrange to have an interpreter present to explain procedures and tests.

Evaluation

Evaluation should include feedback from the client and family to determine their reaction to the interventions. Revisions to the plan of care should be made with client and family input, and alternative sources and resources brought in when needed to enhance communication and exchange of information. Nurses should also perform self-evaluations to identify their attitudes toward caring for clients from diverse cultures.

REFERENCES

Estin, P. (1999). Spotting depression in Asian patients. *RN, 62*(4), 39–40.

WELLNESS CONCEPTS

The responsibility for maintaining health rests squarely on the shoulders of each individual adult. Parents are responsible for maintaining their children's health and teaching them a healthy lifestyle. Health maintenance involves the whole person and the person's whole life. It includes the prevention of disease and the early detection and treatment of disease. Maintenance of health requires constant effort and a focus on all aspects of a person's life.

HEALTH

A widely accepted definition of health comes from the World Health Organization (WHO), which defines health as a state of complete physical, mental, and social well-being, not merely the absence of disease or infirmity.

Other concepts of health focus on motivation. Health is the full realization of potential, and illness is an impediment to that realization.

Those who hold the adaptive view of health are motivated by altering the risks in the individual or the environment through such means as dietary and exercise programs or reducing exposure to environmental hazards. Illness results when the individual is unable to cope with the risks and stresses of daily life.

Some individuals are motivated by being able to meet responsibilities at home, at work, at play, and in the community: Their health focus is role performance. Health is considered achieved when the individual fulfills the obligations and responsibilities to family, job, and community.

Other individuals are motivated by the absence of disease: Theirs is a clinical health focus. As long as no disease is present, the individual considers himself healthy. One's personal definition of health influences life choices and personal health decisions.

WELLNESS

Wellness is defined as a state of optimal health wherein an individual moves toward integration of human functioning, maximizes human potential, takes responsibility for health, and has greater self-awareness and self-satisfaction. Researchers outline seven areas of wellness: emotional, mental, intellectual, vocational, social, spiritual, and physical wellness. Various areas of wellness overlap and none is mutually exclusive.

HEALTH PROMOTION

Health promotion means more than preventing illness: It means assisting individuals to enhance their health, well-being, and functioning and to maximize their potential. Health promotion focuses on adopting healthy behaviors rather than on avoiding illness. The goal is for individuals to control and improve their health. Health promotion is appropriate for the individual and the population as a whole.

ILLNESS PREVENTION

Prevention (hindering, obstructing, or thwarting a disease or illness) incorporates both old and new ideas. The taboos, dietary laws, and traditions of various cultural, ethnic, and religious groups were initiated for a reason. If scientific research has not proved these incorrect or harmful, there is no reason not to practice the old ways. New methods of illness prevention emerge as technology expands and health awareness increases.

All stages of life should embody the tenets of preventive health. It must begin before conception with healthy parents and prenatal care and continue through the life span. Scientific advice based on firmly established medical data and reasonable probability should be heeded.

Types of Prevention

Prevention extends to all stages of health. There are three types of prevention: primary, secondary, and tertiary.

Primary Prevention

Primary prevention includes all practices designed to keep health problems from developing. Primary prevention should be the focus for every individual and health care provider. It is usually the least expensive intervention and provides the greatest benefits.

Secondary Prevention

Secondary prevention refers to early detection, diagnosis, screening, and intervention to reduce the consequences of a health problem. That is, disease or illness is identified before the individual has any symptoms or functional impairment. When no known methods of primary prevention exist for a specific disease or illness (such as breast cancer), the focus should be on performing self-examinations, having a regular physical exam, and testing.

Tertiary Prevention

Tertiary prevention refers to caring for a person who already has a health problem; the illness or disease is treated after symptoms have appeared so as to prevent further progression. Rehabilitation is an important aspect of tertiary prevention; this refers to preventing deterioration of a person's condition and minimizing the loss of function.

Prevention Health Care Team

The prevention health care team consists of the individual assisted by nurses and the primary physician.

Individual

The individual is the center of the prevention health care team. It is the individual who must incorporate the knowledge related to preventive health care and make the behavioral changes necessary to live a more healthy life. *The ultimate responsibility for health care belongs with the individual.*

Nurses

Nurses, especially nurse practitioners, often do the initial health screening in clinics and physicians' offices. This provides a great opportunity to inquire about lifestyle and the preventive health habits of the client.

Primary Physicians

Primary physicians generally are family practitioners, pediatricians, or internists: These are the family doctors, the physicians seen on a regular basis. They have the opportunity and obligation to discuss and inquire about preventive health habits. When necessary, they refer clients to specialists for specific problems.

FACTORS AFFECTING HEALTH

A great many factors affect health. They can be categorized into four broad topics:

Genetics and Human Biology

Inherited traits and the way the human body functions have an impact on an individual's state of health and wellness. An individual's genetic makeup may include inherited disorders, such as sickle-cell anemia, or chromosomal anomalies, such as Down syndrome. Both of these may ultimately affect the individual's quality of life and level of health. Human biology affects health because normal body functioning prevents some illnesses and makes us more susceptible to others.

Personal Behavior

Personal behavior is the area having the most factors affecting health and wellness, and they are controlled entirely by the individual. Factors typically deemed to be under the individual's control include diet, exercise, personal care, sexual relationships, level of stress, tobacco and drug use, alcohol use, and safety.

Environmental Influences

Environmental factors that influence health may be natural or man-made, and vary depending on geographic location and living conditions. Natural disasters and extreme weather conditions pose health risks, as do man-made environmental crises.

Health Care

Most people use the health care system when they are ill, for the treatment of their disease or condition.

Table 7–1 CONTROLLABLE FACTORS FOR TOP 10 CAUSES OF DEATH

CAUSE OF DEATH	CONTROLLABLE FACTORS
Heart disease	Tobacco use, high blood pressure, high cholesterol, lack of exercise, excessive stress, diabetes, obesity
Cancer	Tobacco use, radiation, alcohol abuse, improper diet, environmental exposure
Stroke	Tobacco use, high blood pressure, high cholesterol, lack of exercise
Chronic lung disease	Tobacco use, environmental exposures
Accidents	Alcohol abuse, drug abuse, tobacco use, failure to use seat belts, fatigue, stress, recklessness
Pneumonia and influenza	Chronic lung disease, environmental exposures, tobacco use, alcohol abuse, lack of immunization
Diabetes	Obesity, improper diet, lack of exercise, excessive stress
AIDS	Unsafe sex, neglecting condom use
Suicide	Excessive stress, alcohol abuse, drug abuse
Liver disease	Alcohol abuse, exposure to toxins (ingested and environmental), lack of immunizations

Top 10 data from National Center for Health Statistics (1997), Monthly vital statistics report. *45 (11S2) 23, 40–43. [On-line] Available: www.youfirst.com/risks.htm*

A more effective use of the health care system, however, is health promotion and disease prevention. Routine physical examinations with minimal testing and keeping immunizations up-to-date are invaluable for maintaining health and preventing disease. Healthy adults should consider health care services based on factors related to family health history, personal health history, personal habits, or the presence of symptoms that may alter the time frame for suggested health care services.

GUIDELINES FOR HEALTHY LIVING

Because of their education and training, nurses are in a unique position to practice healthy living habits themselves and to promote such habits in their clients. Table 7–1 outlines select causes of death and the controllable lifestyle factors that most contribute to these types of deaths.

REFERENCE

National Center for Health Statistics. (1997). *Monthly vital statistics report, 45*(11S2), 23, 40–43. [On-line] www.youfirst.com/risks.htm

ALTERNATIVE/ COMPLEMENTARY THERAPIES

The use of alternative therapies (therapies used *instead of* conventional or mainstream medical modalities) and complementary therapies (therapies used *in conjunction with* conventional medical therapies) is becoming more prevalent among the general public (Keegan, 1998).

Nurses are encouraged to think critically before recommending or implementing any of these approaches. Whether they simply discuss alternative/complementary therapies with clients or perform these therapies, nurses should understand the ramifications.

Because more and more states are regulating alternative/complementary therapies, nurses must know the laws that govern these therapies in the states in which they work.

Employer policy and the nurse's job description must also be checked to confirm that performing alternative/complementary therapies is within the nurse's scope of practice at that agency. Employer malpractice insurance policies typically do not cover situations where a client is injured as a result of an alternative/complementary therapy.

As holistic caregivers, nurses may employ alternative/complementary techniques to promote clients' well-being. It is important to establish that healing (to make whole) is not the same as curing (ridding one of disease), but is instead a process that activates the individual's forces from within. This means that the nursing assessment must include eliciting information regarding client use of complementary/alternative therapies (Hodge & Ullrich, 1999).

ALTERNATIVE/ COMPLEMENTARY INTERVENTIONS

Many alternative/complementary interventions are used in holistic nursing practice. These interventions are categorized as mind/body, body-movement, energetic-touch, spiritual, nutritional/medicinal, and other methodologies.

Mind/Body (Self-Regulatory) Techniques

Self-regulatory techniques are methods by which an individual can, independently or with assistance, consciously control some functions of the sympathetic nervous system (for example, heart rate, respiratory rate, and blood pressure). When the client is learning the way to perform these techniques, an assistant is involved; later, however, the client can perform them independently. Self-regulatory techniques include:

- Meditation
- Relaxation
- Imagery
- Biofeedback
- Hypnosis

Body-Movement (Manipulation) Strategies

Body-movement therapies employ techniques of moving or manipulating various body parts to achieve therapeutic outcomes. Modalities include movement and exercise, yoga, tai chi, and chiropractic treatment.

Energetic-Touch Therapies

Many energetic-touch therapies are being used by nurses today. Touch, therapeutic massage, therapeutic touch, and healing touch are some examples. Other modalities include acupressure and reflexology, techniques that involve deep-tissue body work and require advanced training on the part of practitioners.

Touch

One of the most universal alternative/complementary modalities is touch. It should be noted that touch carries with it taboos and prescriptions that are culturally dictated. Some cultures are very comfortable with physi-

cal touch; others specify that touch may be used only in certain situations and within specified parameters.

Because touch involves personal contact, the nurse must be sure to convey positive intentions. When in doubt, the nurse should withhold touch until effective communication with the client has been established.

It may be difficult for persons who have been neglected, abused, or injured to accept touch therapy. Touching those who are distrustful or angry may escalate negative behaviors. Persons with burns or overly sensitive skin may not benefit from touch.

Therapeutic Massage

Therapeutic massage is the application of pressure and motion by the hands with the intent of improving the recipient's well-being. Massage therapy is now recognized as a highly beneficial modality and is prescribed by a number of physicians. In addition, many states now have licensing requirements for massage practitioners.

Back rubs have been administered by nurses to provide comfort to hospitalized clients. Massage techniques can be used with all age groups and are especially beneficial to those who are immobilized. A back rub or massage can achieve many results, including relaxation, increased circulation of the blood and lymph, and relief from musculoskeletal stiffness, pain, and spasm.

Massage should never be attempted in areas of circulatory abnormality, such as aneurysm, varicose veins, necrosis, phlebitis, or thrombus, or in areas of soft-tissue injury, open wounds, inflammation, joint or bone injury, dermatitis, recent surgery, or sciatica.

Therapeutic Touch

Therapeutic touch, which is based on ancient healing practices such as the laying on of hands, consists of assessing alterations in a person's energy field and using the hands to direct energy to achieve a balanced state.

Healing Touch

Healing touch is an energy-based therapeutic modality that alters the energy field through the use of touch.

Shiatsu and Acupressure

Shiatsu, from the word meaning "finger pressure," is a Japanese form of acupressure. Acupressure is a technique of releasing blocked energy within an individual when specific points (Tsubas) along the meridians are pressed or massaged by the practitioner's fingers, thumbs, and heels of the hands. When the blocked energy is freed, the disease subsides.

Reflexology

The foot is viewed as a microcosm of the entire body. The pressing of specific points on the foot stimulates energy movement and produces relaxation, reduces stress, and promotes health by relieving pressure and accumulation of toxins in the corresponding body part.

Spiritual Therapies

A state of wholeness or health is dependent on one's relationship not only to the physical and interpersonal environments, but also to the spiritual aspects of self. The role of the spirit in healing is witnessed in all cultures.

Faith Healing

This process, based on religious belief, is usually accomplished through prayer. During preparation for healing, the practitioner adapts a passive and receptive mood in order to be a channel for divine power. The ill person's belief enhances, but is not crucial to, the success of healing.

Healing Prayer

When individuals pray, they believe they are communicating directly with God or a Higher Power. Prayer is an integral part of a person's spiritual life and, as such, can affect well-being.

Nutritional/Medicinal Therapies

In the past 20 to 30 years, nutritional interventions for prevention and treatment of disease have generated increasing interest among consumers and health care providers.

Phytochemicals

Phytochemicals are plant chemicals that have several functions including storage of nutrients and provision of structure, aroma, flavor, and color. They are found in fruits and vegetables. Nurses can use this information to encourage clients to eat more fruits and vegetables.

Herbal Therapy

Many drugs commonly used today were, in an earlier time, tribal remedies derived from plants. Herbs work because of their chemical composition. Different herbs contain different compounds that can strengthen the immune system, alter the blood chemistry, or protect specific organs against disease.

Others

S-adenosylmethionine (SAMe) is a modified amino acid produced naturally by the body; however, the level decreases with age. Controlled research has shown that SAMe may benefit clients with osteoarthritis.

Omega-3 fatty acids, found in salmon, trout, sardines, walnuts, canola oil, and flax seeds help reduce the threat of cardiac arrhythmias. Research has also shown that the omega-3 fatty acids suppress inflammation of rheumatoid arthritis and may improve glucose control in type 2 diabetes.

Other Methodologies

Other methodologies such as aromatherapy, humor, pet therapy, music therapy, and play therapy are also used.

Aromatherapy

Aromatherapists use concentrated oils derived from the roots, bark, or flowers of herbs and other plants to treat specific ailments. Some essential oils have antibacterial properties and are found in a wide variety of pharmaceutical preparations. Essential oils are very potent and should never be used in an undiluted form, be used near the eyes, or be ingested orally. Because some people are allergic to certain oils, a small skin patch test should be done before generalized application.

Humor

Humor is the intervention that can be used most often by nurses to benefit clients. To avoid giving offense, it is important to determine the client's perception of what is humorous. Whether a given situation is considered humorous or offensive will vary greatly from culture to culture and person to person. Good taste and common sense should serve as guides.

Nurses can use humor with clients in a variety of ways. A humor cart (portable cart or carrier filled with cartoon and joke books, magic tricks, and silly noses) is easy to use and allows clients to select their own humor tools for health. A "humor room" may be made available, where clients can watch comedy videos or play fun games with visitors or other clients.

Humor can be used effectively to relieve anxiety and promote relaxation, improve respiratory function, enhance immunological function, and decrease pain by stimulating the production of endorphins.

Pet Therapy

Pet therapy is used as treatment for people in both acute and long-term care settings. There are many applications including overcoming physical limitations, improving mood, lowering blood pressure, and improving socialization skills and self-esteem.

Music Therapy

Therapeutic use of music consists of playing music to elicit positive changes in behavior, emotions, or physiological response. Music complements other treatment modalities and encourages clients to become active participants in their health care and recovery.

Music on audiocassette and heard via a tape player and headphones can be a very useful tool for clients who are immobilized, who must wait for diagnostic tests, or who are undergoing the perioperative experience. Some facilities allow clients to choose the type of music played while they undergo procedures such as cardiac catheterization. Clients may request that their music and tape player accompany them during surgery. Pleasurable sound and music can reduce stress, perception of pain, anxiety, and feelings of isolation. Music can also be especially useful in helping adolescent clients relax.

Play Therapy

Toys are used to allow children to learn about what will be happening to them and to express their emotions and their current situations. Drawing and artwork also provide a way for children to share their experiences.

NURSING AND ALTERNATIVE/ COMPLEMENTARY APPROACHES

Nurses play an important role in educating consumers about nontraditional interventions appropriate throughout the life cycle by providing information about the safety and efficacy of such methods.

REFERENCES

Hodge, P., & Ullrich, S. (1999). Does your assessment include alternative therapies? *RN, 62*(6), 47–49.

Keegan, L. (1998). Alternative & complementary therapies. *Nursing98, 28*(4), 50–53.

LOSS, GRIEF, AND DEATH

Nurses must be aware of the potential for loss in today's world, as well as the processes whereby individuals react and adapt to losses. Many people consider loss only in terms of death and dying; however, loss of every type occurs daily. Grief is a response to losses of all types.

LOSS

Loss is any situation, either actual, potential, or perceived, wherein a valued object or person is changed or is no longer accessible to the individual. A loss can be tangible or intangible. For example, when a person is fired from a job, the tangible loss is income, whereas the loss of self-esteem is intangible.

GRIEF

Grief, a series of intense physical and psychological responses that occur following a loss, is a normal, natural, necessary, and adaptive response to a loss. Loss leads to the adaptive process of mourning, the period of time during which grief is expressed and resolution and integration of the loss occur. Bereave-

ment is the period of grief following the death of a loved one.

Types of Grief

Grief is a universal, normal response to loss. Grief drains people, both emotionally and physically. There are different types of grief, including uncomplicated ("normal"), dysfunctional, anticipatory, and disenfranchised grief.

Nurses with a sound knowledge base of both normal grief and dysfunctional grief are better prepared to assist survivors than are nurses who mistakenly believe that all grief is the same.

Uncomplicated Grief

Uncomplicated grief is what many individuals would refer to as *normal grief.*

Dysfunctional Grief

Dysfunctional grief is a demonstration of a persistent pattern of intense grief that does not result in reconcilation of feelings. The person is unable to adapt to life without the deceased.

Anticipatory Grief

Anticipatory grief is the occurrence of grief work before an expected loss actually occurs. Anticipatory grief may be experienced by the terminally ill person as well as the person's family. This phenomenon promotes adaptive grieving and, therefore, frees up the mourner's emotional energy for problem solving.

Disenfranchised Grief

Grief can become disenfranchised when an individual either is reluctant to recognize the sense of loss and develops guilt feelings or feels pressured by society to "get on with life."

Factors Affecting Loss and Grief

The following variables may possibly affect the intensity and duration of grieving:

- Developmental stage
- Religious and cultural beliefs
- Relationship with the lost object
- Cause of death

Nursing Care of the Grieving Client

Resolution of a loss is a painful process and must be done by clients in their own way. Nurses can assist by providing support as the client moves through the process of mourning.

Nurses can play an active role in assisting people to grieve by encouraging clients to do their grief work, that is, to experience their feelings to the fullest in order to work through them.

Providing support and explaining to the bereaved that it will take time to grieve the loss and to gain some closure to the relationship are both important nursing responsibilities.

Assessment

A thorough assessment of the grieving client and family begins with a determination of the personal meaning of the loss. Another key assessment area is deciding the person's progress in terms of the grieving process. The stages of grieving are not necessarily mastered sequentially.

Nursing Diagnosis

Two nursing diagnoses may be appropriate: *Dysfunctional Grieving* and *Anticipatory Grieving* (NANDA, 2001).

Planning/Outcome Identification

Listed below are some expected goals for the person experiencing grief:

- Verbalize feelings of grief
- Share grief with significant others
- Accept the loss
- Renew activities and relationships

Implementation

Therapeutic nursing care is based on an understanding of the significance of the loss to the client. The nurse's nonjudgmental, accepting attitude is essential during the bereaved's expression of all feelings, including anger and despair. Grieving people need reassurance, counseling, and support. One mechanism of support on a long-term basis is support groups.

Evaluation

People follow their own time schedule for grief work. In general, it takes months or years for grief resolution. The nurse has a unique opportunity to lay the foundation for adaptive grieving by encouraging the bereaved to share their feelings and to continue to verbalize their experience with significant others.

DEATH

Just as each person lives a unique life, each person dies a unique death. Health care workers must understand the legal and ethical issues surrounding dying and death. Nurses must also come to terms with their own mortality and feelings about death if they are to provide comfort to dying clients and their families.

Legal Considerations

According to the *Patient Self-Determination Act* (PSDA), all clients entering the health care system through hospitals, long-term care facilities, home health agencies, hospice programs, and some health maintenance organizations, must be given information and the opportunity to complete advance directives if they have not already done so. The medical record must have a written do-not-resuscitate (DNR) order from a physician if this is in agreement with the client's wishes and with the advance directives. In the absence of such an order, resuscitation will be initiated.

Nursing Care of the Dying Client

The death process is typically a very emotional time for clients and their families; compassionate and sensitive nursing care that respects clients' wishes as well as meets their physical needs can help bring peace and dignity to this natural process.

Assessment

Assessment of the dying client includes an ongoing collection of data regarding the strengths and limitations of the dying person and the family.

Nursing Diagnoses

The nurse's assessment of the dying client may lead to any number of diagnoses. NANDA-approved nursing diagnoses that are applicable for many dying clients are *Powerlessness* and *Death Anxiety.*

Planning/Outcome Identification

The dying client must be treated as a unique individual worthy of respect, rather than as a diagnosis to be cured. Many dying clients do not fear death but are anxious about a painful death or dying alone.

Promoting optimal quality of life means treating the client and family in a respectful manner and providing a safe environment for the expression of feelings. Planning focuses on meeting the holistic needs of the client and family. In planning care, the nurse should make every effort to be sensitive to the dying client's rights.

Implementation

The nurse's first priority is to communicate a caring attitude to the client. Terminally ill clients are often given palliative care, or care that relieves symptoms, such as pain, but does not alter the course of disease. A primary aim of palliative care is to help the client feel safe and secure. The nurse can do much to increase the client's feelings of safety by being available when needed. Holding the client's hand and listening are therapeutic measures.

PHYSIOLOGICAL NEEDS Areas that are often problematic for the terminally ill client are respirations; fluids and nutrition; mouth, eyes, and nose; mobility; skin care; and elimination.

Respirations Oxygen is frequently ordered for the client experiencing labored breathing. Suctioning may be needed to remove secretions that the client is unable to swallow.

Fluids and Nutrition The refusal of food and fluids is almost universal in dying clients. It is believed that the client is not feeling thirst and hunger.

Mouth, Eyes, and Nose Oral discomfort is the only documented side effect of dehydration in the terminally ill client (Taylor, 1995). Use saliva substitutes and moisturizers to alleviate discomfort. Offer ice chips and sips of favorite beverages and apply petroleum jelly to the lips.

The eyes may become irritated due to dryness. Artificial tears can alleviate this discomfort.

A thin layer of water soluble jelly applied to the nares will help alleviate discomfort.

Mobility As the client's condition deteriorates, mobility decreases. The client should be repositioned at least every 2 hours.

Skin Care The prevention of pressure ulcers is a priority. Regular repositioning and passive range of motion exercises are two preventive measures. Keeping the skin clean and moisturized will promote healthy tissue.

Elimination Constipation may occur due to side effects of pain medications and to lack of physical activity.

The client may become incontinent of bladder and bowel, so the nurse must check the client frequently, clean the skin with peri-washes, and apply a moisture barrier after each incontinent episode.

Comfort The primary activities directed at promoting physical comfort include pain relief, keeping the client clean and dry, and providing a safe, nonthreatening environment.

Physical Environment A soothing physical environment can significantly increase the client's comfort.

PSYCHOSOCIAL NEEDS Death presents a threat to not only one's physical existence, but to one's psychological integrity.

For many clients, maintaining a well-groomed appearance is important. Caregivers should presume that the client would prefer to maintain the same grooming habits as were previously preferred.

SPIRITUAL NEEDS Nurses play a major role in promoting the dying client's spiritual comfort.

Some therapeutic nursing interventions that address the spiritual needs of the dying client include:

• Communicate empathy
• Play music
• Use touch
• Pray with the client
• Contact clergy, if requested by the client
• Read religious literature aloud, at the client's request

SUPPORT FOR THE FAMILY Family members need to be involved in the care of their dying loved one. Each family member will grieve the approaching death in her own way. The nurse must be supportive and nonjudgmental.

Impending Death

Even when death is expected, it is never easy for the family. The family should be thoroughly informed, in simple terms, about what will happen before and after the client's death, including:

• Physical changes that will occur just before and following death
• Pronouncement of death
• Post-mortem care
• Removal of the body

Secretions accumulate in the larynx and trachea, causing noisy respirations, often called the "death rattle."

The heart fails in its pumping function, resulting in poor perfusion, ischemia, and cell death. The skin becomes cool and, possibly, very pale, cyanotic, jaundiced, or mottled. The pulse becomes rapid, irregular, weak, and thready. Death is several hours away if a peripheral pulse is strong and easily palpated. Cold, cyanotic extremities and irregular respirations indicate that death may be expected within an hour or two (Durham & Weiss, 1997).

The care of the client does not cease during this final stage of life. The nursing actions previously described should be continued. The nurse should tell the client in brief, simple terms what is happening as care is rendered. The family should be allowed and encouraged to continue their participation, if that is their wish. The nurse should caution family members that *the dying client can hear even in the absence of verbal response,* so all comments and conversation should continue to be respectful.

Care after Death

Caring for the deceased body and meeting the needs of the grieving family are nursing responsibilities. Post-mortem care is given immediately after death but before the body is moved to the mortuary.

In preparing the body for family viewing, the nurse strives to make the body look comfortable and natural. The nurse is also responsible for returning the deceased's possessions, such as jewelry, eyeglasses, clothing, and all other personal items, to the family.

Legal Aspects

It is important for nurses to know their legal responsibilities, which are defined by their respective state boards of nursing.

Autopsy

An unexpected death and a violent death are circumstances that would necessitate an autopsy. Families must give consent for an autopsy to be performed in other situations. The funeral director must know whether an autopsy is to be performed.

Organ Donation

It is important that families of the deceased know the need for and process of organ donation.

When the family gives consent for donation, the donor team is notified that an organ is available for transplant. Time is of the essence, because the organ or tissue must be harvested and transplanted quickly to maintain viability.

Care of the Family

The nurse provides information about viewing the body, asks the family about donating organs, and offers to contact support people (e.g., other relatives, clergy). Sensitive and compassionate interpersonal skills are essential in providing information and support to families.

REFERENCES

Durham, E., & Weiss, L. (1997). How patients die. *AJN, 97*(12), 41–46.

Taylor, M. (1995). Benefits of dehydration in terminally ill clients. *Geriatric Nursing, 16*(6), 271–272.

AREAS OF MEDICAL-SURGICAL NURSING CARE

FLUID, ELECTROLYTE, AND ACID–BASE BALANCE

Our bodies must continually adjust to changes in the external environment. In order for life to continue, however, our internal environment—the one inside our bodies—must remain relatively constant, varying only slightly within narrow ranges. Constant maintenance of the internal environment within very narrow limits—in equilibrium—is termed homeostasis.

HOMEOSTASIS

Homeostasis is an ongoing process; that is, the body simply does not reach a state of equilibrium and remain there. When the body loses the ability to maintain homeostasis, and the internal environment changes, the physiologic processes can be interrupted or changed, leading to disease, disorder, or death. Maintaining homeostasis is essential to life.

WATER

Water is so integral to the body's processes that fluctuations in the amount of water in the body can have harmful or even fatal consequences.

FLUID AND ELECTROLYTE BALANCE

For life to continue and the cells to properly function, the body fluids must remain fairly constant with regard to the amount of water and the specific electrolytes of which they are composed. Water is essential because it is the basic component of all the body fluids.

Body Fluids

The major ions in the extracellular fluid are sodium (Na^+), chloride (Cl^-), and bicarbonate (HCO_3^-), although other ions do occur. In the intracellular fluid, the major ions are potassium (K^+), phosphate (PO_4^{--}), and magnesium (Mg^{++}), with lesser amounts of other ions present. There are also large numbers of protein molecules bearing a negative charge.

Exchange between the Extracellular and Intracellular Fluids

Water and ions moving between the extracellular and intracellular fluids must first pass through the selectively permeable cell membrane. This movement is governed primarily by osmosis. If the amount of interstitial fluid returned to the circulatory system lessens and the fluid accumulates in the tissue spaces, the tissues become swollen. This condition is called edema. A number of conditions can cause edema, including kidney or liver disease and heart disorders.

When more water is lost from the body than is replaced, dehydration occurs. Among the various causes of dehydration are water deprivation, excessive urine production, profuse sweating, diarrhea, and extended periods of vomiting.

Regulators of Fluid and Electrolyte Balance

There must be a balance in the amounts of fluids and electrolytes consumed and lost daily. Under typical conditions, the average adult loses some water through the skin, lungs, and GI tract and loses the largest amount of water through urine production. This can amount to a per-day fluid loss of approximately 2500 mL, depending on conditions.

Fluid and Food Intake

Fluids must be replaced in the amounts lost. The primary source of fluid replacement is water consumption. Approximately 60% may be obtained in this way, with an additional 30% being obtained from foods and 8% to 10% being a product of metabolism (metabolic water) for a total of 2,500 mL.

Thirst

Water consumption usually occurs in response to the sensation of thirst.

One nursing goal is to ensure that all clients understand both the role that water plays in health and the way to maintain adequate hydration.

DISTURBANCES IN ELECTROLYTE BALANCE

In illness, one or more of the regulating mechanisms may be affected, or an imbalance may become too great for the body to correct without treatment.

Sodium

Sodium (Na^+) is the major electrolyte in extracellular fluid. Excretion occurs primarily via the kidneys. The normal serum sodium for an adult is 136 to 145 mEq/L.

Potassium

Potassium (K^+) is the major electrolyte in intracellular fluid. Its concentration inside cells is approximately 150 mEq/L. The normal value range of extracellular (serum) potassium is narrow: 3.5 to 5.0 mEq/L. Consequently, the slightest changes can dramatically affect physiological functions.

When replacing potassium chloride:

- Use IV route only when hypokalemia is life threatening or when oral replacement is not feasible
- Always dilute potassium chloride in a large amount of IV solution
- Never administer more than 10 mEq/L of IV potassium chloride (KCl) per hour; the normal dose of IV KCl is 20 to 40 mEq/L infused over an 8-hour period

- Never give KCl intramuscularly (IM) or as an IV bolus; potentially fatal hyperkalemia may result
- Monitor the IV site frequently for early signs of infiltration, as potassium is caustic to the tissues

Calcium

Calcium (Ca^{++}) plays an essential role in bone and teeth integrity, blood clotting, muscle functioning, and nerve impulse transmission. The normal ionized serum calcium range for an adult is 4.5 to 5.6 mEq/L. Total serum calcium concentration measures both the ionized calcium and the calcium bound to albumin. The normal value range of total serum calcium concentration for an adult is 9.0 to 10.5 mg/dL, with values for the older adult being slightly lower. Approximately 50% of serum calcium is bound to protein. Correlate the serum calcium level with the serum albumin level when evaluating laboratory results. *Any change in serum protein will result in a change in the total serum calcium.*

Magnesium

Most magnesium (Mg^{++}) is found in intracellular fluid and in combination with calcium and phosphorus in bone, muscle, and soft tissue. Blood serum contains only approximately 1%. A close relationship exists among magnesium, calcium, and potassium in the intracellular fluid: A low level of one results in low levels of the other two. The normal serum magnesium level for an adult is 1.5 to 2.5 mEq/L.

Phosphate

Phosphate (PO_4^{--}) is the main intracellular anion. It appears as phosphorus in the serum, where the normal value range is 1.7 to 2.6 mEq/L. Phosphorus is critical for normal cell functioning.

Chloride

Chloride (Cl^-) is the major anion in extracellular fluid. Chloride functions in combination with sodium to maintain osmotic pressure. It also assists in maintaining acid–base balance. The normal serum chloride range is 95 to 106 mEq/L.

ACID–BASE BALANCE

A pH below 7.35 is termed acidosis, and a pH above 7.45 is termed alkalosis. Either of these conditions can be brought about by respiratory or metabolic changes.

Regulators of Acid–Base Balance

The body has three main control systems that regulate acid–base balance to counter acidosis or alkalosis: the buffer systems, respirations, and renal control of hydrogen ion concentration. These systems vary in their reaction times in regulating and restoring balance to the hydrogen ion concentration.

Buffer Systems

The buffer systems—bicarbonate, phosphate, and protein—react quickly to prevent excessive changes in the hydrogen ion concentration.

Respiratory Regulation of Acid–Base Balance

The respiratory system helps to maintain acid–base balance by controlling the content of carbon dioxide in extracellular fluid.

It takes the respiratory regulatory mechanism several minutes to respond to changes in the carbon dioxide concentration of extracellular fluid.

Renal Control of Hydrogen Ion Concentration

The kidneys control extracellular fluid pH by eliminating either hydrogen ions or bicarbonate ions from body fluids. The renal mechanism for regulating acid–base balance cannot readjust the pH within seconds; but it can function over a period of several hours or days to correct acid–base imbalance.

Diagnostic and Laboratory Data

The biochemical indicators of acid–base balance are assessed by measuring the arterial blood gases (ABGs). The arterial blood gas test measures the levels of oxygen and carbon dioxide in arterial blood. The test assesses pH, partial pressure of oxygen (PO_2 or PaO_2), partial pressure of carbon dioxide (PCO_2 or $PaCO_2$), saturation of oxygen (SaO_2), and bicarbonate (HCO_3).

The PO_2 or PaO_2 expresses the amount of oxygen that can combine with hemoglobin to form oxyhemoglobin, the form in which oxygen is transported through the body. At sea level, the normal range is 80 to 100 millimeters of mercury (mm Hg).

The PCO_2 or $PaCO_2$ in the blood is a reflection of the efficiency of gaseous exchange in the lungs. At sea level, the normal range is 35 to 45 mm Hg.

The SaO_2 is the percent of oxygen that combines with hemoglobin in the blood. The normal range is 95% to 100% saturation. Oxygen saturation can also be measured with a pulse oximeter, a noninvasive technique. Warming a client's cold hand will provide more accurate results from a pulse oximeter.

Determining the amount of bicarbonate (HCO_3) in the blood is important because, along with carbonic acid, bicarbonate is a major buffer in the blood. The two substances occur in a ratio of 20 parts bicarbonate to 1 part carbonic acid. Regardless of the carbonic acid and bicarbonate values, the pH of the blood will remain in the normal range as long as the ratio remains 20:1. The normal range for HCO_3 at sea level is 24 to 28 mEq/L. The carbonic acid level is always 3% of the PCO_2 level.

DISTURBANCES IN ACID–BASE BALANCE

The acid–base imbalances are respiratory acidosis and alkalosis and metabolic acidosis and alkalosis. In determining whether the acid–base imbalance is caused by a respiratory or a metabolic alteration, the key indicators are bicarbonate and carbonic acid levels. Table 10–1 lists those changes in laboratory values that indicate the various acid–base imbalances.

Respiratory Acidosis

When carbon dioxide is not eliminated by the lungs as fast as it is

Table 10-1 LABORATORY VALUES IN ACID–BASE IMBALANCES

SITUATION	PH	PCO$_2$	HCO$_3$
Normal parameters	7.35 to 7.45	35 to 45 mm Hg	24 to 28 mEq/L
Respiratory acidosis			
Acute	< 7.35	> 45 mm Hg	Normal
Chronic	< 7.35	> 45 mm Hg	> 28 mEq/L
Respiratory alkalosis	> 7.45	< 35 mm Hg	Normal
Metabolic acidosis	< 7.35	Normal	< 24 mEq/L
Metabolic alkalosis	> 7.45	Normal	> 28 mEq/L

produced by cellular metabolism, the amount of carbon dioxide increases in the blood. It then reacts with water and forms excess hydrogen ions. It is caused by hypoventilation or any condition that depresses ventilation.

Clients with respiratory acidosis experience neurological changes resulting from the acidity of the cerebrospinal fluid and brain cells. Hypoventilation causes hypoxemia (decreased oxygen in the blood), which in turn causes further neurological impairment. Hyperkalemia may accompany acidosis.

Respiratory Alkalosis

Respiratory alkalosis is characterized by a decreased hydrogen ion concentration (a blood pH above 7.45) and a below normal PCO$_2$ level (lower than 35 mm Hg). It is caused by hyperventilation (excessive exhalation of carbon dioxide) resulting in hypocapnia (decreased arterial carbon dioxide concentration). As the breathing returns to normal, the carbon dioxide level in the blood in-

creases, and the normal pH is restored.

Metabolic Acidosis

Metabolic acidosis is characterized by an increase in hydrogen ion concentration (blood pH below 7.35) or a decrease in bicarbonate concentration. Such a change may be brought about by kidney disease when the mechanism to excrete excess hydrogen ions is compromised. Diarrhea, diabetes mellitus, and, sometimes, diuretics may also be responsible. Metabolic acidosis is most common in individuals with kidney disease or diabetes mellitus.

Metabolic Alkalosis

Metabolic alkalosis is characterized by a loss of acid from the body or a gain in base (increased level of bicarbonate). Excessive oral or parenteral administration of sodium bicarbonate or other alkaline salts (e.g., sodium or potassium acetate, lactate, or citrate) increases the amount of base in extracellular fluid. Loss of gastric fluids from vomiting or suctioning may result in metabolic alkalosis.

The rate and depth of respirations decrease in an effort to retain carbon dioxide. To counter the pH imbalance of metabolic alkalosis, the arterial carbon dioxide concentration rises, creating respiratory acidosis.

NURSING PROCESS

The nursing process assists the nurse in planning client care.

Assessment

Electrolyte and acid–base imbalances are identified primarily with laboratory data, while a fluid imbalance is identified primarily with the health history and physical examination.

Physical Examination

DAILY WEIGHT Changes in the body's total fluid volume are reflected in body weight. For instance, each liter (1,000 mL) of fluid gained or lost is equivalent to 1 kilogram (2.2 lb) of weight.

VITAL SIGNS An elevated temperature places the client at risk for dehydration related to an increased loss of body fluid.

Changes in the pulse rate, strength, and rhythm are indicative of fluid alterations:

- Fluid volume deficit: increased pulse rate and weak pulse volume
- Fluid volume excess: increased pulse volume and third heart sound

Changes in the respiratory rate and depth may cause respiratory acid–base imbalances or may be indicative of a compensatory response to metabolic acidosis or alkalosis.

Fluid volume deficit can lower the blood pressure. A narrow pulse pressure (lower than 20 mm Hg) may indicate fluid volume deficit that occurs with severe hypovolemia.

INTAKE AND OUTPUT A minimum intake of 1,500 mL is essential in balancing urinary output and the body's insensible water loss.

SKIN Edema and skin turgor are two important indicators related to fluid, electrolyte, and acid–base balances.

Edema is the main symptom of fluid volume excess. The body may retain 5 to 10 pounds of fluid before edema is noticeable (Bulechek & McCloskey, 1999). The dependent body parts—sacrum, back, and legs—should be assessed for peripheral edema. Pitting edema is rated on a four-point scale, as follows:

+0: no pitting
+1: 0 to ¼ inch pitting (mild)
+2: ¼ to ½ inch pitting (moderate)
+3: ½ to 1 inch pitting (severe)
+4: greater than 1 inch pitting (severe)

Dehydration is the main cause of decreased skin turgor, which manifests as lax skin that returns slowly to the normal position. Increased skin turgor manifests as smooth, taut, shiny skin that cannot be grasped and raised.

BUCCAL (ORAL) CAVITY   With fluid volume deficit, saliva decreases, causing sticky, dry mucous membranes and dry, cracked lips. The tongue displays longitudinal furrows.

EYES   Inspect the eyes for sunkenness, dry conjunctiva, and decreased or absent tearing—all signs of fluid volume deficit. Puffy eyelids (periorbital edema, or papilledema) are characteristic of fluid volume excess.

JUGULAR AND HAND VEINS   Circulatory volume is assessed by measuring venous filling of the jugular and hand veins.

NEUROMUSCULAR SYSTEM   Fluid and electrolyte imbalances may cause the muscles to lose their tone and become soft and flabby, and reflexes to diminish. Calcium and magnesium imbalances cause an increase in neuromuscular irritability. Other neurological signs of fluid, electrolyte, and acid–base imbalances include inability to concentrate, confusion, and emotional lability.

Diagnostic and Laboratory Data

Laboratory tests can reveal imbalances before clinical symptoms are evident in the client. However, unless clients are having the tests for some other reason, symptoms are detected first.

Nursing Diagnosis

The primary nursing diagnoses for clients with fluid imbalances are *Excess Fluid Volume, Deficient Fluid Volume, Risk for Deficient Fluid Volume,* and *Risk for Imbalanced Fluid*

Volume. Numerous secondary nursing diagnoses may also apply.

Excess Fluid Volume

Excess Fluid Volume exists when the client has edema and increased interstitial and intravascular fluid retention. Fluid volume excess is related to excess fluid in either the tissues of the extremities (peripheral edema) or the lung tissues (pulmonary edema).

Assessment findings in the client with fluid volume excess include acute weight gain; decreased serum osmolality (lower than 275 mOsm/Kg), protein and albumin, blood urea nitrogen (BUN), Hgb, Hct; increased central venous pressure (greater than 12 to 15 cm H_2O); and signs and symptoms of edema. The clinical manifestations of edema are relative to the area of involvement, either pulmonary or peripheral.

Deficient Fluid Volume

Deficient Fluid Volume exists when the client experiences vascular, interstitial, or intracellular dehydration. The degree of dehydration is classified as mild, marked, severe, or fatal on the basis of the percentage of body weight lost.

Assessment findings in the client with fluid volume deficit include thirst and weight loss. Marked dehydration manifests as dry mucous membranes and skin; poor skin turgor; low-grade temperature elevation; tachycardia; respirations of 28 or greater; decreased (10 to 15 mm Hg) systolic blood pressure; slowed venous filling; decreased urine output (fewer than 25 mL/hr); concentrated urine; elevated Hct, Hgb, and

BUN; and acidic blood pH (less than 7.4).

Severe dehydration is characterized by the symptoms of marked dehydration plus a flushing of the skin. Systolic blood pressure continues to drop (to 60 mm Hg or below), and behavioral changes (restlessness, irritability, disorientation, and delirium) occur. The signs of fatal dehydration are anuria and coma leading to death.

Risk for Deficient Fluid Volume

Risk for Deficient Fluid Volume exists when the client is at risk of developing vascular, interstitial, or intracellular dehydration resulting from active or regulatory loss of body water in excess of needs.

Risk for Imbalanced Fluid Volume

Risk for Imbalanced Fluid Volume exists when the client is at risk for a decrease, increase, or rapid shift from one to the other of intravascular, interstitial, and/or intracellular fluid. This refers to body fluid loss, gain, or both.

Planning/Outcome Identification

Holistic nursing care for clients experiencing a fluid imbalance requires that the nurse, in collaboration with each client, identify specific goals for each nursing diagnosis. Expected outcomes for the client with a fluid imbalance are not only specific to the primary diagnosis, but also must be relative to the interventions.

Implementation

The rationale for interventions related to alterations in either fluid, electrolyte, or acid–base balance is based on the goal of maintaining homeostasis and regulating and maintaining essential fluids and nutrients. The most common interventions include:

- Monitor daily weight
- Measure vital signs
- Measure intake and output
- Provide oral hygiene
- Initiate oral fluid therapy—Oral fluids may be totally restricted—a situation commonly referred to as *nothing by mouth* (NPO)—or they may be restricted or forced, depending on the client's clinical situation.
- Maintain tube feeding—When the client cannot ingest oral fluids but has a normal GI tract, fluids and nutrients can be administered through a feeding tube as prescribed by a physician.
- Monitor intravenous therapy

Evaluation

The focus of evaluation should be on the client's responses. The client's vital signs should be within normal limits. The IV infusion rate should be accurately calculated and reassessed throughout therapy to maintain the client's hydration. The IV site should remain free from erythema, edema, and purulent drainage.

REFERENCE

Bulechek, G., & McCloskey, J. (1999). *Nursing interventions: Effective nursing treatments* (3rd ed). Philadelphia: W. B. Saunders.

IV THERAPY

IV therapy administration requires specialized knowledge, judgment, and nursing skills.

INTRAVENOUS THERAPY

Intravenous (IV) therapy is the administration of fluids, electrolytes, nutrients, or medications by the venous route. It requires parenteral fluids (solutions) and special equipment: administration set, IV pole, filter, regulators to control IV flow rate, and an established venous route.

PARENTERAL FLUIDS

The nurse should confirm the type and amount of IV solution by reading the physician's order in the client's medical record. Intravenous solutions are sterile and are packaged in plastic bags or glass containers. Solutions that are incompatible with plastic are dispensed in glass containers.

Plastic IV solution bags collapse under atmospheric pressure to allow the solution to enter the infusion set. When the plastic solution bag is removed from its outer wrapper, the solution bag should be dry. If the solution bag is wet, the nurse should not use the solution. The moisture on the bag indicates that the integrity of the bag has been compromised and that the solution cannot be considered sterile. The bag should be returned to the dispensing department that issued the solution. Glass containers are discussed in the section on equipment.

EQUIPMENT

Intravenous equipment is sterile, disposable, and prepackaged with user instructions. The syringe tip and port require sterile technique during handling because they are in direct contact with fluids to be infused into the bloodstream. The protective caps keep both ends of the infusion set sterile and are removed only just before use. The insertion spike is inserted into the port of the IV solution container.

Nonvented infusion sets are used with plastic bags of IV solutions and vented bottles. The vented set is used for glass containers that are not vented.

There are two types of drip chambers: a macrodrip, which delivers 10 to 20 drops per milliliter of solution, and a microdrip, which delivers 60 drops per milliliter. The drip rate, which is indicated on the package, varies with the manufacturer.

PREPARING AN INTRAVENOUS SOLUTION

To prepare an IV solution, the nurse should first read the agency's protocol and gather the necessary equipment. Because IV equipment and solutions are sterile, the expiration date on the package should be checked before use. The solution can be prepared at the nurses' work area or in the client's room.

Prepare and apply a time strip to the IV solution bag to facilitate monitoring of the infusion rate as prescribed by the physician. The IV tubing is tagged with the date and time to indicate when the tubing replacement is necessary. Intravenous tubing is changed every 24 to 48 hours according to agency policy. The nurse initials the time strip and the IV tubing tag. *Do not use a felt-tip pen to mark an IV bag. The ink from the pen can leak through the plastic and contaminate the solution. Instead, mark a sticker or piece of tape, then affix this to the bag.*

INITIATING IV THERAPY

When initiating IV therapy, first consider the type of fluid to be infused and then assess for a venipuncture site. Ellenberger (1999) suggests that the smallest gauge and shortest needle appropriate be selected (22 gauge for maintenance fluids and routine antibiotics, 20 gauge or larger for blood products). When assessing a client for potential sites, consider age, body size, activity, clinical status and impairments, and skin condition. Generally, it is best to begin with the hand and advance up the arm if new sites are needed. Figure 11-1 illustrates common peripheral sites for initiating IV therapy. Venipuncture site contraindications are:

- Signs of infection, infiltration, or thrombosis
- Affected arm of a postmastectomy client
- Arm with a functioning arteriovenous fistula (dialysis)
- Affected arm of a paralyzed client
- Any arm that has circulatory or neurological impairments

Locating a Vein

With the client's arm extended on a firm surface, place a tourniquet on the arm, tight enough to impede venous flow yet loose enough that a radial pulse can still be palpated. Next,

---

Professional Tip: Inserting a CVC

When assisting with the insertion of a long-line central catheter, observe the client for symptoms of a pneumothorax: sudden shortness of breath or sharp chest pain; increased anxiety; a weak, rapid pulse; hypotension; pallor or cyanosis. These symptoms indicate accidental puncture of the pleural membrane.

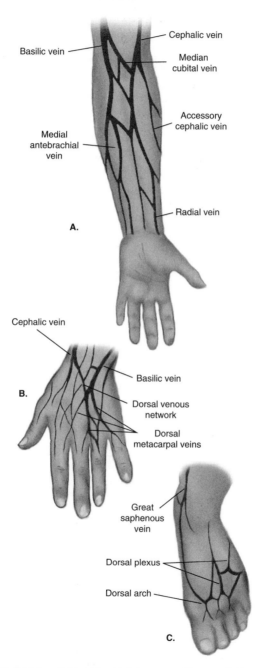

Figure 11-1 Peripheral Veins Used in Intravenous Therapy: A. Forearm; B. Dorsum of the hand; C. Dorsal plexus of the foot

use the index and middle fingers of the nondominant hand to palpate a vein. It should feel soft and resilient and not have a pulse. If no vein can be seen or felt, a warm, moist compress may be applied for 10 to 20 minutes, the area may be massaged toward the heart, or the client may open and close the fist (Ellenberger, 1999).

Placing the Needle

With hands washed and gloved, prepare the selected site according to agency policy. Without touching the prepared site, stabilize the vein by placing your thumb beside the vein and pulling down. Hold the needle at a 10- to 30-degree angle, bevel up to puncture the skin, then lessen the angle to prevent puncturing the back of the vein (Ellenberger, 1999). Secure the needle in place according to agency policy.

When prepping the client's skin for a venipuncture, cleanse the skin with Betadine and wait for it to dry. Do not apply alcohol after the skin has been prepped with Betadine. If these substances are combined, they form a toxic material that may be absorbed through the skin.

ADMINISTERING IV THERAPY

Once the solution has been prepared for administration, calculate the rate and explain the procedure to the client.

Calculating Flow Rate

The flow rate is the volume of fluid to infuse over a set period of time as prescribed by the physician. The physician will identify the amount to infuse per time period such as: 125 mL per hour or 1,000 mL over an 8-hour period. The hourly infusion rate is calculated as follows:

$$\frac{\text{Total volume}}{\text{Number of hours to infuse}} =$$

$$\text{mL/hour infusion rate}$$

For example, if 1,000 mL is to be infused over 8 hours:

$$\frac{1,000}{8} = 125 \text{ mL/hour}$$

Calculate the actual infusion rate (drops per minute) as follows:

$$\frac{\text{Total fluid volume}}{\text{Total time (minutes)}} \times \text{Drop factor}$$

$$= \text{Drops per minute}$$

For example, if 1,000 mL is to be infused over 8 hours with a tubing drop factor of 10 drops per milliliter:

$$\frac{1,000 \text{ mL}}{8 \ (60) \text{ min}} \times 10 \text{ drops/mL} =$$

$$\frac{10,000 \text{ drops}}{480 \text{ min}} = \frac{20.8, \text{ or } 21,}{\text{drops/min}}$$

Another way to calculate the actual infusion rate is to use the hourly infusion rate; for the first example:

$$\frac{125 \text{ mL} \times 10 \text{ drops/mL}}{60 \text{ min}} =$$

$$20.8 \text{ or } 21 \text{ drops/min}$$

Volume Controllers and Pumps

When setting the volume to be infused (e.g., 1,000 mL), set the volume to be infused slightly lower (e.g., 950 mL) so that the alarm will go off before the fluids are completely gone. This practice gives time to have the next bag of fluid ready when all 1,000 mL has be absorbed. Having the extra time is especially helpful when dealing with refrigerated fluids that must be warmed to room temperature before being administered. If you will be off duty when the volume will be absorbed and the alarm is set to go off early, tell the oncoming nurse during report.

INTRAVENOUS DRUG THERAPY

Intravenous administration provides immediate release of medication into the bloodstream; consequently it can be dangerous. Intravenous medications are administered by one of the following methods:

- Intravenous fluid container
- Volume-control administration set
- Intermittent infusion by piggyback or partial fill
- Intravenous push (IVP or bolus)

Adding Drugs to an Intravenous Fluid Container

Before administering any IV medication, note the client's allergies, drug or solution incompatibilities, the amount and type of diluent needed to mix the medication, and the client's general condition to establish a baseline for administering medication. Check for drug compatibilities of drug additives before injecting a medication into an infusion bag.

Administering Medications by Intermittent Infusion

A common method of administering IV medications is by using a secondary, or partial-fill additive bag, often referred to as an IV piggyback (IVPB). A secondary line is a complete IV set (fluid container and tubing with either a microdrip or a macrodrip system) connected to a Y-port of a primary line. The primary line maintains venous access. The IVPB is used for medication administration. When the IVPB medication is incompatible with the primary IV solution, the nurse must flush the primary IV tubing with normal saline before and after administering the medication.

Administering IV Push Medications

The method of medication administration by IV push (bolus) injection is determined by the type of IV system. For example, an IV push medication can be injected into a saline or a heparin lock or into a continuous infusion line. When giving an IV push medication into a continuous infusion line, the nurse must stop the fluids in the primary line by pinching the IV tubing closed while injecting the drug. This technique is safe and prevents the nurse from having to recalculate the drip rate of the primary infusion line.

BLOOD TRANSFUSION

When the physician prescribes the administration of whole blood or a blood product, the client's blood is typed and crossmatched. Check with the family for donors if time and the client's condition permit. The blood is stored in the blood bank after typing and crossmatching.

Although whole blood has a refrigerated shelf life of 35 days, platelets must be administered within 3 days after they have been extracted from whole blood.

Initial Assessment and Preparation

The nurse must perform an initial assessment before administering blood. The nurse should:

- Verify that the client has signed a blood administration consent form and that this consent matches what the physician has prescribed.
- Verify whether the client has an 18- or a 19-gauge needle or catheter in a vein. The viscosity of whole blood usually requires this gauge needle or catheter to prevent damage to the red blood cells. If blood is to be infused quickly, a 14- or 15-gauge device must be used.
- Ensure patency of the existing IV site.
- Establish baseline data for vital signs, especially temperature, and assess skin for eruptions or rashes.
- Check client's blood type against the label on the whole blood or blood component before administration, to ensure compatibility.
- Assess the client's age and state of nutrition.
- If elderly clients are at risk for circulatory overload, notify the blood bank to divide the 500-mL bag of blood into two 250-mL bags or discuss with the physician other alternatives, such as packed RBCs rather than whole blood.

Scheduled IV medications should be infused before blood administration. This sequence prevents a reaction to a medication while blood is infusing. If a reaction were to occur, the nurse would not be able to discern whether the medication or the blood was causing the reaction.

Administering Whole Blood or a Blood Component

The agency's blood protocol may require that a licensed person sign a form to release the blood from the blood bank and that a blood product be checked by two licensed personnel before infusion. The following information must be on the blood bag label and verified for accuracy: the client's name and identification number, ABO group and Rh factor, donor number, type of product ordered by the practitioner, and expiration date.

Only normal saline should be used with a blood product. Blood transfusions are incompatible with dextrose and with Ringer's solution.

Blood should be administered within 30 minutes after it has been received from the bank, to maintain RBC integrity and to decrease the chance of infection. Whole blood should not go unrefrigerated for more than 4 hours. Room temperature will cause RBC lysis, releasing potassium and causing hyperkalemia.

Safety Measures

The client should be observed for the initial 15 minutes for a transfusion

Table 11–1 NURSING ACTIONS FOR BLOOD REACTIONS

IMMEDIATE NURSING ACTION	OTHER MEASURES
• Stop transfusion. • Keep vein open with normal saline. • Notify the physician.	• Monitor client's vital signs every 15 minutes for 4 hours or until stable. • Monitor I&O. • Send IV tubing and bag of blood back to the blood bank. • Obtain a blood and urine specimen. • Label specimen "Blood Transfusion Reaction." • Process a transfusion reaction report.

reaction. Vital signs are usually taken every 15 minutes for the first hour, then every hour while the blood is transfusing.

There are three basic types of transfusion reactions: allergic, febrile, and hemolytic. Other complications include sepsis, hypervolemia, and hypothermia. An allergic reaction may be mild or severe, depending on the cause. Hemolytic reactions may be immediate or delayed up to 96 hours, depending on the cause of the reaction. The classic symptoms of a reaction and sepsis are fever and chills. The severity of a transfusion reaction is relative to its onset. Severe reactions may occur shortly after the blood starts to infuse. At the first sign of a reaction, stop the blood infusion immediately.

The nursing actions for all types of reactions and complications are given in Table 11–1.

REFERENCE

Ellenberger, A. (1999). Starting an IV line. *Nursing99, 29*(3), 56–59.

HEALTH ASSESSMENT

Nursing assessment includes both physical and psychosocial aspects to evaluate a client's condition. A thorough nursing assessment includes both a health history and a physical examination. Other sources of objective data are laboratory tests, x-rays, and measurements of the client's vital signs, height, and weight.

HEALTH HISTORY

A primary focus of the data collection interview is the health history. The health history is a review of the client's functional health patterns prior to the current contact with a health care agency. Included in the health history are the following:

- Demographic information
- Reason for seeking health care
- Perception of health status
- Previous illnesses, hospitalizations, and surgeries
- Client/family medical history
- Immunizations/exposure to communicable diseases
- Allergies
- Current medications
- Developmental level

- Psychosocial history
- Sociocultural history
- Alternative/complementary therapy use
- Activities of daily living
- Review of systems

PHYSICAL EXAMINATION

The physical examination is performed in all health care settings (home, outpatient facilities, extended care institutions, and acute care facilities) for all age groups to gather comprehensive, pertinent assessment data. The physical examination provides a complete picture of the client's physiological functioning. When combined with a health and psychosocial assessment, it forms a database to direct decision making. The examination should be performed according to the agency's policy. Policy may vary from one agency to another.

It is performed in a sequential, head-to-toe fashion to ensure a thorough assessment of each system. Specific assessment techniques include:

- Inspection
- Palpation

- Percussion
- Auscultation

This method not only prevents the nurse from forgetting to examine an area, it also decreases the number of times the nurse and the client have to change positions.

HEAD-TO-TOE ASSESSMENT

The client's privacy should be respected by pulling the curtain, closing the door, and providing appropriate draping of the client. When possible, distracting noises such as radio or television and people talking should be eliminated. Assessment should be performed under natural light because fluorescent light can change the color tones of the skin. All procedures should be explained to the client and confidentiality of data acquired during the examination maintained.

Standard precautions should be utilized when in contact with any body fluids by using gloves, gown, or mask when appropriate.

General Survey

It is important for the nurse to identify herself and to express intent for the care of the client and the time frame involved. During this introductory time, it is appropriate for the nurse to utilize inspection to make a general assessment of the client. It is important to consider clients in the context of their cultural beliefs.

Elderly Clients

When nurses assess elderly clients, it is important to know the normal changes that result from aging.

Clients with Disabilities

Adapt interactions to the client's ability. To allay the client's fears and anxiety, a family member may be allowed to remain with the client during the examination.

Clients Who Are Abused

Observe for signs of abuse, especially in the elderly. The symptoms may include refusal to be touched, inability to maintain eye contact, or unwillingness to talk about bruises, burns, or other injuries. The nurse must know state laws and agency policies for reporting possible abuse.

Vital Signs

When checking vital signs, the nurse obtains the temperature, pulse, respirations, and blood pressure of the client.

Temperature

Consumption of hot or cold food or beverage and smoking 15 to 30 minutes before taking an oral temperature can affect the result.

To convert Fahrenheit to Celsius (centigrade):

$$(\text{Temperature } °F - 32) \times 5/9 = °C$$

Example:

$$98.6°F - 32 = 66.6 \times 5/9 = 37°C$$

To convert Celsius to Fahrenheit:

$$9/5 \times \text{temperature}°C + 32 = °F$$

Example:

$$9/5 \times 40°C = 72 + 32 = 104°F$$

Pulse

The most accessible peripheral pulses are the radial and carotid sites. Because the body shunts blood to the brain whenever a cardiac emergency such as hemorrhage occurs, the carotid site should always be used to assess the pulse in these situations. When assessing a carotid pulse, apply light pressure to only one carotid artery to avoid disruption of cerebral blood flow. Then assess the other one.

Respirations

Normal breathing is slightly observable, effortless, quiet, automatic, and regular. It can be assessed by observing chest wall expansion and bilateral symmetrical movement of the thorax. Each respiration includes one complete inhalation (breathing in) and exhalation (breathing out) by the client.

Blood Pressure

The most common site for indirect blood pressure measurement is the client's arm over the brachial artery. When the client has any of the following, *do not* measure blood pressure on the involved side:

- Venous access devices, such as an intravenous infusion or arteriovenous fistula for renal dialysis
- Surgery involving the breast, axilla, shoulder, arm, or hand
- Injury or disease to the shoulder, arm, or hand, such as trauma, burns, or application of a cast or bandage

Height and Weight Measurement

Measuring height and weight is as important as assessing the client's vital signs.

Height

The metal rod attached to the back of the scale should be extended to gently rest on the top of the client's head, and the measurement should be read at eye level.

Weight

When a client has an order for "daily weight," the weight should be obtained at the same time of day on the same scale, with the client wearing the same type of clothing. The client should wear some type of light foot covering, such as socks or disposable operating room slippers, to prevent the transmission of infection and to enhance comfort.

Head and Neck Assessment

Head and neck are assessed to determine the client's mental and neurological status, and the client's overall affect (outward expression of mood or emotion), as well as physical attributes.

Hair and Scalp

The hair and scalp of a client should be inspected. The hair distribution, quantity, texture, and color should be noted. The scalp should be smooth and free of any debris or infestations.

Eyes

The eyes should be symmetrical. Check the eyebrows and eyelids to determine if there is any drooping, which may be a sign of muscle weakness or neurological impairment. The color of the sclera and conjunctiva, as well as the presence of any drainage, should be noted. The pupils should be assessed to determine their size, shape, and reaction to light.

Nose

The nose should be symmetrical, midline, and in proportion to other features. Any deformity, inflammation, or prior trauma should be noted.

Lips and Mouth

The lips and mucous membranes of the mouth are observed for color, symmetry, moisture, or lesions. Unusual breath odors should be noted.

Neck

The neck should be assessed to determine if there is full range of motion, for any enlargement of the lymph nodes or thyroid gland, and for any pulsations in the neck. The carotid pulsation is seen just below the angle of the jaw. Normally there are no other visible pulsations while the client is in the sitting position.

Mental and Neurological Status and Affect

A client's mental status includes identification of the level of orientation to person, place, and time.

Neurological assessment of the client focuses on the following: level of consciousness (LOC), pupil response, hand grasps, and foot pushes.

Skin Assessment

Assessment of the skin should be performed as each area of the body is assessed. The color of the skin as well as its moisture or dryness, temperature, turgor, edema, and integrity, should be noted.

The location, size, distribution, and appearance of skin lesions throughout the body are described. Scratches, bruises, skin tears, cuts, and scars from previous injuries or surgeries are noted.

Thoracic Assessment

During thoracic assessment, the nurse will determine the condition of the client's cardiovascular and respiratory systems along with assessment of the breasts.

Cardiovascular Status

Assessment of the client's cardiovascular status by the LP/VN focuses specifically on listening to the apical pulse, comparing peripheral pulses bilaterally, identifying heart tones, and checking the nail beds and skin color. Ask if the client has ever fainted or felt dizzy. Any lower leg swelling and its cause should also be noted.

Respiratory Status

Breath sound assessment is performed after determination of the apical pulse rate. Respiratory auscultation reveals the presence of normal and abnormal breath sounds. During auscultation of breath sounds, the client should be instructed to breathe only through the mouth because mouth breathing decreases air turbulence that could interfere with an accurate assessment.

Ask the client about any difficulty breathing or the presence of a cough (nonproductive or productive), and to describe the secretions produced.

Wounds, Scars, Drains, Tubes, Dressings

Note any type of wounds, scars, drains, tubes, or dressings the client may have. Assessment of these must include the location, size, and amount of drainage or discharge, and if present, signs of inflammation.

Breasts

Assessment of the breast tissue should be done for both male and female clients. Note if the client has had mammography and when the last x-ray was taken.

Abdominal Assessment

During abdominal assessment, the nurse determines the status of the client's gastrointestinal and genitourinary systems. Note any type of wounds, scars, drains, tubes, dressings, or ostomies the client may have. Because palpation can affect sounds heard on auscultation, the sequence for abdominal assessment is as follows:

- Inspection
- Auscultation
- Percussion
- Palpation

Gastrointestinal Status

The abdomen is first inspected for rashes and scars and if the abdomen is flat, rounded, or distended. Auscultation is the second component of the abdominal assessment of a client's bowel status. A "bubbly-gurgly" sound should be heard in all four quadrants of the abdomen. When approximately 5 to 20 bowel sounds are heard per minute, or 1 at least every 5 to 15 seconds, the bowel sounds are considered active.

After assessment of bowel sounds, the nurse should question the client about diet, usual bowel patterns, appetite, weight changes, indigestion, heartburn, nausea, pain, and use of enemas or laxatives.

Genitourinary Status

Assessment of the client's urinary and reproductive status is accomplished mainly by inspection and use of interview skills. Genitourinary assessment includes examination of the abdomen, urinary meatus and genitalia, and assessment of the client's urine. Ask about any history of urinary tract infections, kidney stones, change in the urinary stream, or painful urination or nocturia.

Musculoskeletal and Extremity Assessment

Hand grasps and foot pushes assess the strength and equality of the client's extremities. examination of muscles should occur in pairs, first one extremity and then the other; equality of size, con-tour, tone, and strength should be assessed. Check legs to determine color changes, loss of feeling or hair, change in temperature within the extremity and from one extremity to the other, and presence of varicose veins, ulcers, and edema. Ask the client if muscle weakness is experienced or if difficulty or pain when walking or performing routine daily activities occurs.

SUGGESTED READING

Andresen, G. (1998). Assessing the older patient. *RN, 61*(3), 46–55.

DIAGNOSTIC TESTS

The role of the nurse is to teach the client, family, and significant others about the procedures involved in diagnostic testing, the steps to be taken in preparation for the specific test(s) in question, and the care that will follow the procedure. Although the primary focus is on teaching, the nurse may assist in performing various noninvasive and invasive procedures.

DIAGNOSTIC TESTING

Diagnostic testing is a critical element of assessment. Ongoing client assessment and evaluation of the client's expected outcomes require the incorporation of diagnostic findings. To protect your health and safety, as well as that of other health care providers and the client, use Standard Precautions whenever exposure to body fluids is possible.

Preparing the Client for Diagnostic Testing

Table 13–1 outlines a sample protocol of the nursing care to prepare a client for diagnostic testing.

Care of the Client during Diagnostic Testing

Although client care must be individualized according to the specific procedure, general guidelines for client care during a procedure are outlined in Table 13–2.

Care of the Client after Diagnostic Testing

Postprocedure nursing care is directed toward restoring the client's prediagnostic level of functioning (Table 13–3).

Table 13–1 PROTOCOL: PREPARING THE CLIENT FOR DIAGNOSTIC TESTING	
Purpose	To increase the reliability of the test by providing client teaching on the reason the test is being performed, those things the client can expect during the test, and the outcomes and side effects of the test
	To decrease the client's anxiety about the test and the associated risks
Supportive Data	Increase the client's knowledge, thereby promoting cooperation and enhancing the quality of the testing
	Decrease the time required to perform the tests, thereby increasing cost effectiveness
	Prevent delays by ensuring proper physical preparation
Assessment	Ensure that the client is wearing an identification band
	Review the medical record for allergies and previous adverse reactions to dyes and other contrast media; a signed consent form; and the recorded findings of diagnostic tests relative to the procedure
	Assess for the presence, location, and characteristics of physical and communicative limitations or preexisting conditions
	Monitor the client's knowledge of both the reasons for the test and those things to expect during and after testing
	Monitor vital signs of the client who is scheduled for invasive testing, to establish baseline data
	Assess client outcome measures relative to the practitioner's preferences for preprocedure preparations
	Monitor level of hydration and weakness for clients who are designated nothing by mouth (NPO)
Report to Practitioner	Notify practitioner of allergy, previous adverse reaction, or suspected adverse reaction following the administration of drugs
	Notify practitioner of any client or family concerns not alleviated by discussions with nurse
Interventions	Clarify with practitioner whether regularly scheduled medications are to be administered
	Implement NPO status, as determined by the type of test
	Administer cathartics or laxatives as denoted by the test's protocol; instruct clients who are weak to call for assistance to the bathroom
	Teach relaxation techniques, such as deep breathing and imagery
	Establish intravenous (IV) access if necessary for the procedure

(continues)

Table 13-1 *(continued)*	
Evaluation	Evaluate the client's knowledge of those things to expect
	Evaluate the client's anxiety level
	Evaluate the client's level of safety and comfort
Client Teaching	Discuss the following with the client and family, as appropriate to the specific test:
	• The reason for the test and those things to expect
	• An estimation of how long the test will take
	• Specifics of NPO status, including amount of water to drink if oral medication is to be taken
	• Cathartics or laxative: amount, frequency
	• Sputum: cough deeply, do not clear throat
	• Urine: voided, clean-catch specimen; timing of collection
	• Removal of objects (e.g., jewelry or hair clips) that will obscure x-ray film
	• Contrast medium:
	Barium: taste, consistency, after effects (lightly colored stools for 24 to 72 hours; possibly, obstruction/impaction)
	Iodine: metallic taste, delayed allergic reaction (itching, rashes, hives, wheezing and breathing difficulties)
	• Positioning during the test
	• Positioning posttest (e.g., immobilize limb after angiography)
	• Posttest (encourage fluid intake if not contraindicated)
Documentation	Record in the client's medical record:
	• Practitioner notification of allergies or suspected adverse reaction to contrast media
	• Presence, location, and characteristics of symptoms
	• Teaching and the client's response to teaching
	• Responses to interventions (client outcomes)

Table 13-2 PROTOCOL: CARE OF THE CLIENT DURING DIAGNOSTIC TESTING

Purpose	To increase cooperation and participation by allaying the client's anxiety
	To provide the maximum level of safety and comfort during a procedure
Supportive Data	Encourage relaxation of the muscles and thus facilitation of instrumentation by increasing the client's participation and comfort
	Ensure both efficient use of time during the test and reliable results from the test with proper preparation of the client
Assessment	Check the client's identification band to ensure the correct client
	Review the medical record for allergies
	Assess the client's reaction to the preprocedure sedatives administered prior to the induction of anesthesia during the procedure
	Assess airway maintenance and gag reflex, if a local anesthetic is sprayed into the client's throat
	Assess vital signs throughout the procedure and compare to baseline data
	Assess the client's ability to maintain and tolerate the prescribed position
	Assess the client's comfort level to ensure the effectiveness of the anesthetic agent
	Assess for related symptoms indicating complications specific to the procedure (e.g., accidental perforation of an organ)
Report to Practitioner	Notify the practitioner of any client concerns or questions not answered in discussions with the nurse
	Notify the practitioner of any family members present and their location during the procedure
	Notify the practitioner when the client is positioned properly and the anesthetic agent has been administered to the client
Interventions	Institute Standard Precautions or appropriate aseptic technique for the specific test
	Report to all personnel involved in the test any known client allergies
	Place the client in the correct position, drape, and monitor to ensure that breathing is not compromised
	Remain with the client during induction and maintenance of anesthesia
	If the procedure requires the administration of a dye, ensure that the client is not allergic to the dye; if the client has not received the dye before, perform the skin allergy test according to the manufacturer's instructions that accompany the medication

(continues)

Table 13-2 *(continued)*

Maintain the client's airway and keep resuscitative equipment available

Assist the client to relax during insertion of the instrument by telling the client to breathe through the mouth and to concentrate on relaxing the involved muscles

Explain what the practitioner is doing so that the client knows what to expect

Label and handle the specimen according to the type of materials obtained and the testing to be done

Report to the practitioner any symptoms of complications

Secure client transport from the diagnostic area

Posttest in the diagnostic area:

- Assist the client to a comfortable, safe position
- Provide oral hygiene and water to clients who were designated NPO for the test, if they are alert and able to swallow
- Remain with the client awaiting transport to another area

Evaluation	Evaluate the client's ventilatory status and tolerance to the procedure
	Evaluate the client's need for assistance
	Evaluate the client's understanding of what was performed during the procedure
	Evaluate the client's understanding of findings identified during the procedure
	Evaluate the client's knowledge of what to expect after the procedure
Client Teaching	Discuss the following with the client and family, as appropriate to the specific test:
	• Those things that occurred during the procedure
	• Questions and concerns of the client or family member
	• Those things to expect during the immediate recovery phase
	• Those things to report to the nurse during the immediate recovery phase
Documentation	Record in the client's medical record:
	• Person who performed the procedure
	• Reason for the procedure
	• Type of anesthesic, dye, or other medications administered
	• Type of specimen obtained and where it was delivered
	• Vital signs and other assessment data such as client's tolerance of the procedure or pain/discomfort level
	• Any symptoms of complications
	• Person who transported the client to another area (designate the names of persons who provided transport and the destination)

Table 13–3 PROTOCOL: CARE OF THE CLIENT AFTER DIAGNOSTIC TESTING	
Purpose	To restore the client's prediagnostic level of functioning by providing care and teaching relative to both those things the client can expect after a test and the outcomes or side effects of the test
Supportive Data	Decrease client anxiety by increasing the client's participation and knowledge of expected outcome measures after a diagnostic test
	Through proper postprocedure care and client teaching, alert the client to those signs and symptoms that must to be reported to the practitioner
Assessment	Check the identification band and call the client by name
	Assess the client closely for signs of airway distress, adverse reactions to anesthesic or other medications, and other signs that may indicate accidental perforation of an organ
	Assess for bleeding those areas where a biopsy was performed
	Assess the client's color and skin temperature
	Assess vascular access lines or other invasive monitoring devices
	Assess the client's ability to expel air, if air was instilled during a gastrointestinal test
	Assess the client's knowledge of those things to expect during the recovery phase
Report to Practitioner	Notify the practitioner of any signs of respiratory distress, bleeding, or changes in vital signs; adverse reactions to anesthetic, sedative, or dye; and other signs of complications
	Notify the practitioner of any client or family concerns or questions not answered in discussions with the nurse
	Notify the practitioner when any results are obtained from the diagnostic test
	Notify the practitioner when the client is fully alert and recovered (for an order to discharge)
Interventions	Implement the practitioner's orders regarding the postprocedure care of the client
	Institute Standard Precautions or surgical asepsis as appropriate to the client's care needs
	Position the client for comfort and accessibility so as to facilitate performance of nursing measures
	Monitor vital signs according to the frequency required for the specific test

(continues)

Table 13–3 *(continued)*

	Observe the insertion site for hematoma or blood loss; replace pressure dressing, as needed
	Monitor the client's urinary output and drainage from other devices
	Enforce activity restrictions appropriate to the test
	Schedule client appointments as directed by the practitioner
Evaluation	Evaluate the client's respiratory status, especially if an anesthetic agent was used
	Evaluate the client's tolerance of oral liquids
	Evaluate the client's understanding of the procedural findings of when the practitioner expects to receive written results
	Evaluate the client's knowledge of those things to expect after discharge
Client Teaching	Based on client assessment and evaluation of knowledge, teach the client or family about the following:
	• Dietary or activity restrictions
	• Signs and symptoms that should be reported immediately to the practitioner
	• Medications
Documentation	Record in the client's medical record on the appropriate forms:
	• Assessment data, nursing interventions, and achievement of expected outcomes
	• Client or family teaching and demonstrated level of understanding
	• Written instructions given to the client or family members

PAIN MANAGEMENT

Pain is a phenomenon that crosses all specialties of nursing. No matter the setting, the nurse will be exposed to challenges in pain management.

DEFINITIONS OF PAIN

McCaffery and Pasero (1999) say it best by defining pain as "whatever the person experiencing it says it is, existing whenever [he or she] says it does." The American Pain Society (APS) stresses the importance of self-report: "Pain is always subjective. . . . The clinician must accept the patient's report of pain" (1999).

PURPOSE OF PAIN

Pain serves an important purpose as a protective mechanism. Pain is also useful as a diagnostic tool. Characteristics of the pain, such as the quality and duration, can give important clues in determining a client's medical diagnosis.

FACTORS AFFECTING THE PAIN EXPERIENCE

McCaffery and Pasero (1999) point out that *the client is the only authority*

about the existence and nature of his or her pain. Many factors account for the differences in clients' individual responses to pain, including:

- Age
- Previous experience with pain
- Drug abuse
- Cultural norms

NURSING PROCESS

The nursing process will provide the correct framework for managing a client's pain.

Assessment

Assessment of the client's pain is a crucial function of the nurse. During the assessment process, nurses need to be aware of their own values and expectations about pain behaviors.

Subjective Data

Determine a client's pain threshold and pain tolerance level. The client's description of the pain should cover several qualifiers, including its location, onset and duration, quality, intensity (Figure 14-1), aggravating factors (variables that worsen the pain, such as exercise, certain foods, or

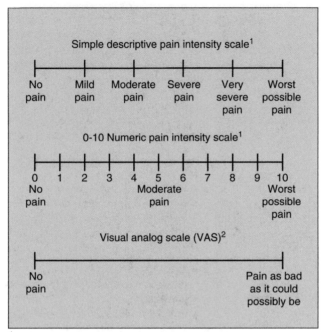

¹ If used as a graphic rating scale, a 10-cm baseline is recommended.
² A 10-cm baseline is recommended for VAS scales.

Figure 14-1 Pain Intensity Scales: Three Commonly Used Self-Report Intensity Scales *(Courtesy of Agency for Health Care Policy and Research, 1992)*

stress), alleviating factors (measures the client can take that lessen the effect of the pain, such as lying down, avoiding certain foods, or taking medication), associated manifestations (factors that often accompany the pain, such as nausea, constipation, or dizziness), and what pain means to the client.

Whenever subjective and objective data conflict, the subjective reports of pain are to be considered the primary source.

Objective Data

Objective data includes physiologic and behavioral data.

PHYSIOLOGIC The client may exhibit the following: elevated heart rate, elevated respiratory rate, elevated blood pressure, diaphoresis, pallor, muscle tension, and dilated pupils. These signs resemble those of anxiety, which often accompanies acute pain. The signs and symptoms of chronic pain show adaption, and, therefore, are different from those of acute pain, with vital signs being normal and no accompanying pupil dilation or perspiration.

BEHAVIORAL Acute pain behaviors may include crying and moaning, rubbing the site of pain, restlessness, a distorted posture, clenched fists, guarding the painful area, frowning, and grimacing. The client usually speaks of the discomfort and may be restless or afraid to move.

The client in chronic pain may demonstrate behaviors similar to those of depression such as hopelessness, listlessness, and loss of libido and weight. Chronic pain also often leads to physical inactivity or immobility, which can lead to functional disability.

Clients often minimize the pain behaviors they are able to control for a number of reasons including:

- To be a "good" client and avoid making demands
- To maintain a positive self-image by not becoming a "sissy"
- By using distraction as a method of making pain more bearable (young children are particularly adept at this)
- Exhaustion

Occasionally, there is a discrepancy between pain behaviors observed by the nurse (objective data) and the client's self-report of pain. Whenever these discrepancies occur, they should be addressed with the client, and the pain management plan must be renegotiated accordingly.

Ongoing Assessment

Pain assessments should be performed to coincide with when the intervention should be providing the most relief.

Recording Pain Assessment Findings

No matter which pain assessment tool is chosen, it will be of little effect unless the pain rating and related information are recorded in a manner easily understood by the health care team.

Nursing Diagnoses

The two primary nursing diagnoses used to describe pain are *Acute Pain* and *Chronic Pain.*

Planning/Outcome Identification

Both nonpharmacologic and pharmacologic interventions should be considered in planning strategies to return clients to control or to maintain them at desired levels of functioning and pain.

Often several approaches must be combined for adequate relief to be obtained. No matter which type of intervention is being utilized, there are three general principles that apply:

- Individualize the approach
- Use a preventive approach
- Use a multidisciplinary approach

Nursing Interventions

Pharmacologic and nonpharmacologic interventions can both be effective in caring for clients with pain. There are three categories of pain control interventions: (1) pharmacological, (2) noninvasive, and (3) invasive. These methods are often used in combination.

Pharmacological Interventions

Drug therapy is the mainstay of treatment for pain control.

NURSES' ROLE IN ADMINISTRATION OF ANALGESICS When analgesics are prescribed, the nurse is often given choices of drug, route, and interval. The nurse must:

- Determine whether or not to give the analgesic, and if more than one is ordered, which one
- Assess the client's response to the analgesic, including assessing the effectiveness in pain relief and occurrence of any side effects
- Report to the physician when a change is needed, including making suggestions for changes based on the nurse's knowledge of the client and pharmacology
- Teach the client and family regarding the use of analgesics

The key to administering an analgesic is to monitor the client's response to it. This includes assessing the effectiveness of pain relief and the occurrence of side effects.

ALTERNATIVE DELIVERY SYSTEMS Opioids are administered in more than just the traditional oral, subcutaneous, intramuscular, intravenous, and rectal routes.

Patient-Controlled Analgesia Patient-controlled analgesia (PCA) is most often delivered by a device that allows the client to control the delivery of intravenous, epidural, subcutaneous, or oral pain medication in a safe, effective manner. This system helps to eliminate the time required for the nurse to provide the medication, and allows the client to feel some control over the pain.

Epidural/Intrathecal Analgesia Epidural analgesia refers to administering the opioid via a catheter that terminates in the epidural space.

Transdermal Analgesia Another route of opioid administration is the transdermal patch. The only opioid drug currently available via this route is fentanyl (Duragesic).

Local Anesthesia Local anesthetics are effective for pain management in a variety of settings.

Noninvasive Interventions

Noninvasive relief measures consist of:

COGNITIVE-BEHAVIORAL INTERVENTIONS These methods can not only help influence the level of pain, but also help the client gain a sense of self-control.

- Trusting nurse–client relationship
- Relaxation
- Reframing
- Distraction
- Guided imagery
- Humor
- Biofeedback

CUTANEOUS STIMULATION This technique involves stimulating the skin to control pain. It is theorized that by stimulating nerve fibers that send signals to the dorsal horn of the spinal cord to "close the gate," pain is relieved. These techniques are not usually meant to replace analgesic therapy, but to complement it.

- Heat and cold application
- Acupressure and massage
- Mentholated rubs
- Transcutaneous electrical nerve stimulation

EXERCISE Exercise is an important treatment for chronic pain because it strengthens weak muscles, helps mobilize joints, and helps restore balance and coordination.

PSYCHOTHERAPY   Psychotherapy may be beneficial to many clients, particularly those:

- In whom the pain is difficult to control
- Who are clinically depressed
- Who have a history of psychiatric problems

POSITIONING   Proper positioning and body alignment minimize exposure to painful stimuli.

Invasive Interventions

Invasive interventions are meant to complement behavioral, physical, and pharmacological therapies. These procedures are usually tried only when noninvasive measures have been attempted first with poor results.

- Nerve Block
- Neurosurgery
- Radiation therapy
- Acupuncture

REFERENCES

Agency for Health Care Policy and Research. (1992). *Clinical practice guideline: Acute pain management: Operative or medical procedures and trauma.* (AHCPR Publication No. 92-0032). Rockville, MD: U.S. Department of Health and Human Services.

American Pain Society. (1999). *Principles of analgesic use in the treatment of acute pain and cancer pain* (4th ed.). Skokie, IL: Author.

McCaffery, M., & Pasero, C. (1999). *Pain: Clinical manual* (2nd ed.). St. Louis, MO: Mosby.

ANESTHESIA

Anesthesia refers to the absence of normal sensation. Analgesia refers to pain relief without producing anesthesia. The delivery of general anesthesia for the purpose of preventing pain during surgery began in the United States in the 1800s. Anesthesia is now a specialty of both nursing and medicine. An anesthesiologist is a licensed physician educated and skilled in the delivery of anesthesia who also adds to the knowledge of anesthesia through research or other scholarly pursuits. An anesthetist is a qualified RN, dentist, or physician who administers anesthetics. The surgical nurse can help prepare clients to talk with their anesthesia providers by encouraging them to ask any questions they have about anesthesia and the care they will receive.

PREANESTHETIC PREPARATION

Preparing a client for anesthesia and surgery is a cooperative effort involving the surgeon, the anesthesia provider, and the nursing staff who will care for the client both before and after surgery.

Oral Intake

Some anesthesia providers prefer that their clients not have anything to eat or drink for at least 8 hours prior to surgery; others may allow water up to 2 hours before. Clearly explain to clients those things that they will or will not be allowed to eat or drink before surgery. Emphasize the need to exactly follow the instructions related to the time at which eating or drinking must cease before surgery.

Preoperative Medication

Exceptions to the practice of continuing scheduled medications prior to surgery include administration of drugs such as insulin and oral antihyperglycemics, nonsteroidal anti-inflammatory drugs (NSAIDs) like aspirin, and anticoagulants like heparin or coumadin.

Additional medications may be ordered to prepare the client for surgery or anesthesia. Some anesthesia providers prefer to give preoperative medications in the operating room to precisely control the medication's effect on the client. This is especially true for very sick clients.

Consent

Consent for anesthesia is usually obtained on the same form as is surgical consent. For an informed consent to be obtained, the anesthetic must be discussed with the client by someone with expert knowledge of anesthesia, usually an anesthesia provider or the surgeon.

Preanesthetic Care

- Complete preoperative checklist.
- Make sure all preoperative orders are executed, especially those for blood tests, preoperative medications, and blood from the blood bank.
- Check, verify, and document the presence or absence of drug allergies for each client.
- Administer regular daily oral medications with a small sip of water as ordered.
- Remind the client of the importance of following instructions regarding any eating or drinking restrictions.
- Administer preoperative medications as close to the ordered time as possible. Timing can be crucial to achieving the desired effect at the correct time.
- If the client responds abnormally to the preoperative medication, notify the anesthesia department immediately.
- Be sure the client's chart is complete when it goes to the operating room with the client. Recent diagnostic test results are especially important to include; otherwise, surgery may be delayed while these results are sought.

- Make sure the client's consents are in order and included in the chart when the client is transported to surgery.

SEDATION AND MONITORING

Sedation is often used to alleviate client anxiety and discomfort during procedures performed under local anesthesia. Because sedatives are CNS depressants and, thus, respiratory depressants, supplemental oxygen should be given to clients during sedation. Monitoring should include an electrocardiogram (EKG), blood pressure, pulse rate, respiratory rate, and continuous oxygen saturation monitoring (pulse oximetry). The individual monitoring the client's breathing and vital signs should be devoted to that task to the exclusion of any other duties.

Residual Effects of Sedation

Amnesia (inability to remember things) produced by sedatives commonly lasts longer than the procedure itself, even in clients who appear to be completely recovered. Such clients will probably not remember any instructions given to them during or soon after the procedure. Given that minor procedures and surgery are commonly performed on an outpatient basis, some clients may be discharged prior to regaining the ability to remember verbal instructions. All instructions should thus be given in writing and explained to the person responsible for taking the client home.

REGIONAL ANESTHESIA

In regional anesthesia a region of the body is temporarily rendered insensible to pain by injection of a local anesthetic.

Types of Regional Anesthesia

There are three types of regional anesthesia: local anesthesia, nerve blocks, and spinal and epidural blocks.

Local Anesthesia

When a small amount of local anesthetic drug is injected either into the skin and subcutaneous tissues around a cut or at the site of a needle puncture for a central line placement, it is called *local anesthesia.*

Topical anesthesia, achieved with direct application of a local anesthetic to tissue, may be desired in some situations. The anesthetic may take the form of an ointment, lotion, solution, or spray. In order to prevent choking and aspiration after the use of an oral anesthetic solution (e.g., viscous lidocaine) or spray, fluids and foods must be withheld until the gag reflex returns.

Nerve Blocks

When a local anesthetic is injected more deeply into the body and/or is directed at a specific nerve or nerves, it is called a *nerve block.*

Spinal and Epidural Blocks

Blocks may also be identified according to where the local anesthetic is injected. One example is an *epidural block,* for which local anesthetic is injected into the epidural space near the spinal cord to anesthetize a number of spinal nerves at once. With *spinal blocks* (also called subarachnoid blocks), the local anesthetic is injected into the cerebrospinal fluid, where it can bathe uninsulated spinal nerves as they exit the spinal cord to the periphery of the body.

When cerebrospinal fluid (CSF) leaks out through a hole made in the dural membrane during performance of a subarachnoid block or an accidental dural puncture during the attempted performance of an epidural block, a postdural puncture headache (PDPH) may result. The headache is relieved by lying down and returns when the individual sits up or stands. The onset of the headache is usually not immediate and may take 1 to 2 days to become bothersome. Treatment involves adequate hydration to allow the normal production of CSF; analgesics; and bed rest in a supine position.

Residual Effects of Regional Anesthesia

All anesthetics must wear off as the drug responsible for causing the anesthesia is removed from its site of action within the body and is metabolized and eliminated. As a regional block begins to wear off, motor function begins to return first, sensation begins to return next, and sympathetic nervous function returns last. Three common residual effects are discussed following.

Residual Motor Block

Any client who has had any type of block involving the legs should never be allowed to get out of bed without assistance until it can be demonstrated that a complete recovery of motor strength in the legs has been regained. Even a small amount of residual motor block greatly increases the possibility that a client will fall.

Residual Sensory Block

As sensation begins to return, the client may experience a "pins and needles" feeling in an arm or leg that has been blocked and may feel touch or pressure before recovering complete sensation. Until complete recovery of normal sensation, any blocked areas of the client's body must be frequently checked and carefully protected, as the client may be unaware that a finger or hand, for example, is being pinched or denied blood supply.

Residual Sympathetic Block

Clients who have had a spinal or epidural block are more likely to have orthostatic hypotension the higher in the spinal column the level of their block. To prevent fainting, clients should not be allowed to get out of bed without the presence of a nurse until after they have been able to do so without any dizziness or significant decrease in blood pressure.

GENERAL ANESTHESIA

General anesthesia involves unconsciousness; complete insensibility to pain; amnesia; motionlessness; and muscle relaxation. With general anesthesia, the body also loses the ability to control many important functions, including the abilities to maintain an airway, control vital functions like breathing and heart rate, and regulate temperature. These functions are controlled by the anesthesia provider during administration of general anesthesia.

Emergence

Emergence from general anesthesia occurs when anesthetic drugs are allowed to wear off. The initial phase of emergence is usually quite quick, allowing the client to awaken enough to respond to verbal directions and maintain an airway. After this time, the client's breathing tube can usually be removed, and the client can be taken to the postanesthesia care unit (recovery room).

Recovery

Recovery from general anesthesia is not complete simply because the client has regained consciousness. The client may not remember what has happened for minutes or even hours after having received an anesthetic. The ability to think clearly often takes longer to return, with some residual thinking difficulty persisting for several days or even weeks.

Oxygenation and Ventilation

Almost all anesthetics are respiratory depressants. Even small amounts of supplemental oxygen given to a client whose rate or depth of breathing is decreased adds significantly to the amount of oxygen in the bloodstream. This is the most important reason that oxygen is given to even healthy clients when they are recovering from general anesthesia.

Temperature Regulation and Shivering

With general anesthesia, the body loses its natural ability to regulate temperature. General anesthetic agents dilate the blood vessels close to the surface of the body, exposing the client's warm blood to the cool exterior. The key to eliminating shivering postoperatively is to ensure client warmth and encourage deep breathing so that the anesthetic is eliminated as quickly as possible.

Fluid Balance

Surgical procedures and the injuries that necessitate them have major effects on the body's distribution of fluid. Large volumes of fluid can be lost to the air through the surgical wound, especially during abdominal procedures. A major abdominal procedure, for example, can result in the loss of up to 10 cc/kg/hour of fluid by evaporation.

POSTANESTHETIC CARE

- Immediately report to the anesthesia provider or surgeon any breathing difficulty.
- Immediately report to the surgeon or the anesthesia department a fall in the client's BP or increase in HR.
- Verify client's ability to stand or walk with normal motor strength and coordination and without any dizziness while in your direct care before allowing the client to get up without assistance.
- Do not allow clients to rub their eyes. Clients who are still drowsy may try to rub out protective eye moisturizer and, in the process, cause painful corneal abrasions.
- Observe clients immediately for bladder distention. Both regional and general anesthesia can sometimes cause temporary urinary retention.
- If clients have an epidural catheter for postoperative pain management, ensure that they change positions from time to time to prevent pressure necrosis. Do not allow the lateral aspect of the leg to rest on the side rails.
- Report to the anesthesia department as soon as possible any headache that gets worse when the client sits up or stands.
- Before giving discharge instructions, verify that the client's ability to remember instructions has returned. Always share discharge instructions with the individual responsible for taking the client home and provide the client with a written copy of the instructions.

NURSING CARE OF THE SURGICAL CLIENT

CHAPTER 16

Regardless of background or roles, surgery is a major stressor for all clients. To a client, there is no such thing as minor surgery; anxiety and fear are normal. Surgery, even when planned well in advance, is a stressor that produces both psychological (anxiety, fear) and physiologic (neuroendocrine) stress reactions. Surgery is a stressful experience because it involves entry into the human body and is sometimes a threat to life itself.

PREOPERATIVE PHASE

The preoperative phase is that time during the surgical experience that begins with the client's decision to have surgery and ends with the transfer of the client to the operating table.

The outcome of surgical treatment is tremendously enhanced by accurate preoperative nursing assessment and careful preoperative preparation. Fear of the unknown is the most prevalent fear prior to surgery and is the fear that the nurse can most easily help control through client education and preoperative teaching.

Preoperative Physiologic Assessment

The nurse's role in preoperative testing is to ensure that the tests are ordered and performed and that the results are placed in the client's chart. Abnormal results are reported to the physician immediately. Tables 16–1 and 16–2 describe topics for client teaching.

INTRAOPERATIVE PHASE

The intraoperative phase is the time during the surgical experience that begins when the client is transferred to the operating room table and ends when the client is admitted to the postanesthesia care unit (PACU).

POSTOPERATIVE PHASE

The postoperative phase is the time during the surgical experience that begins with the end of the surgical procedure and lasts until the client is discharged not just from the hospital or institution, but from medical care by the surgeon. Upon transfer from the operating room, the client usually goes to the PACU.

Table 16-1 TOPICS FOR PREOPERATIVE TEACHING

- Introduce self
    Identify role in client's care
- Determine client's knowledge level and need or desire for additional information
- Explain the routine for the day of surgery
    Restricted food or fluid intake
    Intravenous fluids
    Premedication
    Time of surgery
    Anticipated length of surgery
    Transportation to the operating room
    Special skin preparations
    Type of surgical incision
- Familiarize the client with the operating room environment
    Operating room lights and table
    Accessory equipment
    Monitoring equipment
    Anesthesia induction
- Include significant others
    Time to arrive at the hospital
    Location of surgical waiting area
    What to expect when client returns to the unit
- Explain postanesthesia care unit (PACU)
    Location of recovery room
    Purpose of recovery room
    Routine of postanesthesia care
- Identify anticipated dressings, drains, catheters, casts, etc.
- Demonstrate and evaluate client's proficiency with:
    Coughing and deep breathing exercises
    Turning
    Incentive spirometry
    Extremity exercises
    Any special transfer procedures or aids required after surgery
    See Table 16-2.
- Describe pain management strategies appropriate for the specific surgical
    procedure

Table 16–2	TEACHING POSTOPERATIVE DEEP BREATHING, INCENTIVE SPIROMETRY, COUGHING, AND TURNING	
ACTIVITY	**DESCRIPTION**	**INSTRUCTION**
Deep breathing	• Mode of breathing during which the diaphragm expands fully, allowing expansion of the thorax, upper abdomen, and alveoli as air enters and followed by abdominal and diaphragmatic contraction during expansion	• Sit in semi-Fowler's position with hands placed over lower ribs and upper abdomen • Inhale deeply through the mouth and nose • Hold the breath for 5 seconds • Exhale fully through mouth and nose • Repeat 15 times with short rest periods as needed • Perform twice daily
Incentive spirometry	• Method of using a commercial cylinder that measures deep breaths, with a float that rises during inhalation	• Sit as upright as possible • Seal lips around mouthpiece • Inhale and watch float rise • Hold deep breath for 5 seconds • Remove mouthpiece and exhale slowly • Repeat 10 to 12 times per hour • Cough after the last breath
Coughing	• Method of moving lung secretions from smaller airways to larger airways	• Sit as upright as possible • Splint incision with hands or pillow • Inhale deeply using deep breathing technique • Cough several times until it feels as if no air is left in the lungs • May continue with another deep inhalation followed by one or two strong coughs • Repeat one time per hour

(continues)

Table 16–2 *(continued)*		
ACTIVITY	DESCRIPTION	INSTRUCTION
Turning	• Method of alternating position from back to either side to promote circulation, lung expansion and drainage, and relief from pressure areas	• Change position every 1 to 2 hours (assistance and support pillows may be required)
Leg exercise	• Method of improving circulation in the lower extremities	• Lift leg and circle ankle, first to the right and then to the left. Repeat three times; relax. Repeat with other leg. • With heels on the bed, push toes of both feet toward the foot of the bed until the calf muscles tighten; relax. Pull toes up toward chin until calf muscles tighten; relax feet.

Postoperative Nursing Care

The postanesthesia nurse begins the following nursing assessment and care in the immediate postoperative period:

- Time of arrival in recovery room
- Patency of airway
- Respirations
- Presence of artificial airway devices
  Oral airway
  Nasopharyngeal airway
  Endotracheal airway
- Oxygen saturation
- Need for supplemental oxygen
  Mode of administration
  Flow rate
- Breath sounds
- Color of skin, nail beds, and lips
- Presence of cardiac dysrhythmias

- Other vital signs
  Blood pressure, pulse
- Skin condition (moist or dry, warm or cool) and skin temperature
- Initiate Aldrete Score
- Intravenous infusion
  Type of solution
  Amount in bottle or bag
  Flow rate
  Appearance and location of IV site
- Dressings
  Amount and character of drainage
- Drains and tubes
  Intactness and function
  Connection to drainage and/or suction
  Amount and character of drainage
- Level of consciousness
- Activity level
- Other assessments according to surgical procedure
- Pain

Later Postoperative Nursing Care

Upon the client's arrival in the clinical unit, the nurse assists in the transfer of the client to the bed. Nursing assessment and care of the client upon admission to the clinical unit includes the following:

- Time of arrival in unit
- Transfer from cart to bed
  Place bed in lowest, locked position, with side rails up
  Place client in position of comfort, or as ordered
- Vital signs including airway assessment and breath sounds
- Color of skin, nail beds, and lips
- Skin condition (moist or dry, warm or cool)
- Level of consciousness
- Activity level
- Intravenous infusion
  Type of solution
  Amount in bottle or bag
  Flow rate
  Appearance and location of IV site
- Dressings
  Amount and character of drainage
- Drains and tubes
  Intactness and function
  Connection to drainage and/or suction
  Amount and character of drainage
- Urinary output
  Need to void or time of voiding
  Presence of patency and catheter; output/hour
- Pain
  Last dose of analgesia
  Current pain location, intensity, quality
- Compare assessment with PACU report
- Call light within reach
  Reorient client to usage
- Location of family or significant others
- Postoperative orders

A brief assessment including vital signs is completed every 15 minutes for 1 hour; every ½ hour for 2 hours; and every hour for 4 hours, or as prescribed by physician. The possibilities of postanesthetic complications continue, but as time passes, different postsurgical complications may develop; the nurse is responsible for managing these.

1. *The client is at risk for Ineffective Airway Clearance caused by atelectasis and hypostatic pneumonia.* To prevent these complications, the client is actively encouraged by the nurse to cough, deep breathe (with and without incentive spirometry), and turn as instructed preoperatively. In addition, the client is encouraged to sit up and ambulate as soon and as often as possible.

2. *The client is at risk for Peripheral Neurovascular Dysfunction, Excess/Deficient Fluid Volume, and Activity Intolerance.* The nurse routinely assesses for a positive Homan's sign and for warm, tender, reddened, hardened areas in the calves. The nurse should encourage the client to ambulate to the extent that the client is able. When in bed, the client should perform postoperative leg exercises each hour.

The nurse measures intake and output and monitors laboratory findings (e.g., electrolytes, hematocrit, hemoglobin, and serum osmolality) and signs and symptoms of hemorrhage by assessing vital signs, skin color and condition, dressings, drains, and tubes, as in the PACU.

3. *The client may be at risk for Imbalanced Nutrition: Less than Body Requirements related to nausea and vomiting, hiccoughs, abdominal distension, constipation, and NPO status.* The nurse assesses the client for bowel sounds. After bowel sounds resume in all quadrants, the client may be removed from NPO status according to the surgeon's orders. The nurse also provides good oral hygiene when the client is designated NPO and administers antiemetics as needed for nausea and vomiting.

4. *The client is at risk for developing Urinary Retention related to anesthesia, immobility, and pain. The client is also at risk for Infection related to Foley catheter placement.* Urine output should be at least 30 cc per hour if a catheter is in place.

5. *The client may become at risk for Disturbed Sensory Perception related to anesthesia, narcotics, change of environment, fluid and electrolyte imbalances, sleep deprivation, hypoxia, and sensory deprivation or overload. The client may also experience Acute Pain related to the surgical incision; Hypothermia related to anesthesia and surgical environment; and Hyperthermia related to infection.* Assessing the level of consciousness is a priority. Pain assessment is essential. The nurse's primary role is to prevent infection by using aseptic technique.

6. *The surgical client is at risk for Impaired Skin Integrity and Infection related to surgical incision.* The nurse generally does not remove the primary dressing without an order to do so. In some institutions, the nurse may change the dressing as necessary after the first dressing change. If evisceration occurs, the viscera should be immediately covered with sterile saline dressings and the surgeon notified of the wound disruption.

The major principles to keep in mind when cleansing a surgical incision are:

- Use Standard Precautions at all times.
- Use a sterile swab or gauze and work from the clean area out toward the dirtier area. Begin over the incision line and swab downward from top to bottom. Change the swab and proceed again on either side of the incision, using a new swab each time.

The incisional dressing keeps the incision clean and protects it from physical trauma and bacterial invasion. Generally, the same kind of dressing can be put on as was taken off.

During dressing changes and after the dressing has been removed, the surgical wound is assessed for the skin edge approximation, edema, and bleeding.

7. *Clients are at risk for anxiety or ineffective coping related to disturbance in body image, change in lifestyle, financial strain, or a poor prognosis.* Taking time to talk and listen to the client as well as offering simple explanations

and reassurances may be all the support the client needs to combat anxiety.

As the client recovers and is discharged from the hospital, the client is at risk for knowledge deficit related to home care.

AMBULATORY SURGERY

Ambulatory surgery is defined as surgical care performed under general, regional, or local anesthesia and involving fewer than 24 hours of hospitalization. Today, ambulatory surgery clients are being sent the message that the postoperative client is not sick and, except for a few minor limitations, can often resume normal daily activities soon after undergoing anesthesia and surgery.

ELDERLY CLIENTS UNDERGOING SURGERY

Elderly clients (over 65 years of age) are at risk for developing complications from surgery or anesthesia.

NURSING CARE OF THE ONCOLOGY CLIENT

One in three Americans will develop some type of cancer during their lifetime. Cancer is the second leading cause of death in the United States and can develop in individuals of any race, gender, age, socioeconomic status, or culture.

PATHOPHYSIOLOGY

Cancer is a disease characterized by neoplasia, an uncontrolled growth of abnormal cells. Neoplasms, or any abnormal growth of new tissue, can be found in any body tissue. Neoplasms may be benign (not progressive, and thus, favorable for recovery) or malignant (becoming progressively worse and often resulting in death).

RISK FACTORS

Risk factors, such as environmental, lifestyle, genetic, and viral, may increase an individual's chances of developing cancer.

Environmental Factors

Many industrial chemicals, such as asbestos or vinyl chlorides, have been found to be carcinogenic. The risk of developing cancers is greatly increased if occupational exposure is combined with cigarette smoking.

Lifestyle Factors

Individual lifestyle choices such as the use of tobacco, sun exposure, alcohol consumption, and diet are risk factors.

DETECTION

When cancer does develop, the earlier it is detected the more likely it is to be controlled. A cancer checkup is recommended every 3 years for persons ages 20 to 39 years and annually for those ages 40 years and over.

STAGING OF TUMORS

Staging determines the extent of the spread of cancer. The TNM classification proposed by the American Joint Commission on Cancer is one of the most frequently used systems. The T refers to the anatomical size of the primary tumor; N, the extent of lymph node involvement; and M, the presence or absence of metastasis. Staging is important because it influences decisions about treatment modalities and helps predict overall prognosis.

GRADING OF TUMORS

Grading evaluates tumor cells in comparison to normal cells. Pathologists indicate tumor cell grades by using the Roman numerals I through IV; the higher the grade, the higher the number and the worse the prognosis.

TREATMENT MODALITIES

The most common treatment methods used today are surgery, radiation therapy, and chemotherapy (use of drugs to treat illness); biotherapy and bone marrow transplantation may also be used. These methods may be used alone or in combination.

Surgery

Surgery is the oldest form of cancer treatment and remains the most common method of treatment today.

Radiation Therapy

Radiation therapy, or radiotherapy, uses high-energy ionizing radiation to kill cancer cells.

The goal of radiation therapy is to eradicate malignant cells without causing harm to healthy tissues.

There are two types of radiation therapy: external radiation and internal radiation.

External Radiation

Nursing care should be directed toward client teaching, safety, and carrying out interventions that provide relief from side effects. Client teaching includes:

- Do not wash off the skin markings used to designate reference points for treatment.
- Client is alone in the room during treatment.
- Client must lie absolutely still.
- Treatment typically lasts 1 to 3 minutes.
- Treatment is usually painless.

Undesirable side effects that are most likely to occur include varying degrees of skin reactions and gastrointestinal discomfort such as abdominal cramping, diarrhea, loss of appetite, and fatigue. Treatments have a cumulative effect and may thus produce symptoms after the therapy has been completed.

Internal Radiation

Clients treated with internal sources of radiation can be a source of radioactivity.

When sources are sealed, body fluids are not radioactive. Personnel caring for clients who have sealed sources must still be familiar with the hazards of radiation, however. Generally, the degree of exposure is dependent on three factors:

- The distance between the individual and the source
- The amount of time an individual is exposed
- The type of shielding provided

Some radioactive elements used in unsealed radiation sources are eliminated in body secretions, including urine and stool; thus special precautions should be taken by health care workers to avoid exposure. Agency policies and procedures as well as Standard Precautions must be followed closely. Unsealed sources are not usually radioactive as long as sealed sources are. Nurses should:

- Prepare everything outside of the room so that as little time as possible is spent close to the client;
- Have several nurses assigned to care for the client so that the time of exposure of each nurse is lessened; and
- Wear a lead apron or other shielding device, as provided.

Chemotherapy

Chemotherapy means using chemical therapy or drugs to treat illness, especially cancer. Drugs used in chemotherapy are called antineoplastics because they inhibit the growth and reproduction of malignant cells.

Many of these drugs are given in combination with or after radiation or surgery to achieve maximum effect. The most common routes of administration are oral and intravenous.

Biotherapy

Biotherapy is performed with biologic response modifiers (BRMs), which are agents that stimulate the body's natural immune system to control and destroy malignant cells.

Professional Tip: Chemotherapy and Contamination

- Any personnel handling blood, vomitus, or excreta from clients who have received chemotherapy within the previous 48 hours should wear disposable latex gloves and a disposable gown.
- Place contaminated linen in specially marked laundry bags according to agency procedures.

Professional Tip: Home Care Following Chemotherapy

Teach clients receiving chemotherapy to monitor the side effects of therapy at home.

- Inspect the skin daily for any signs of rash or dermatitis, which may signal hypersensitivity to a drug.
- Report taste loss and tingling in the face, fingers, or toes, which may signal peripheral neuropathy.
- Report signs of dizziness, headache, confusion, slurred speech, or convulsions, which may be signs of central nervous system (CNS) toxicity.
- Report signs of unusual bleeding or bruising; fever; sore throat; or mouth sores, which may signal developing myelosuppression.
- Report signs of jaundice; yellowing of the eyes; clay-colored stools; or dark urine, which may signal developing hepatic dysfunction.
- Report a continued cough or shortness of breath, which may signal developing pulmonary fibrosis.

Bone Marrow Transplantation

Bone marrow transplantation (BMT) is used for cancers that respond to high doses of chemotherapy or radiation therapy. Treatment involves aspirating and storing a fraction of bone marrow, exposing the client to high-dose drug therapy or total body irradiation, and then reinfusing the bone marrow after the treatment is complete.

SYMPTOM MANAGEMENT

One of the most important responsibilities of the oncology nurse is to formulate nursing interventions to manage a variety of secondary problems such as:

- Bone marrow dysfunction
- Nutritional alterations
  1. Anorexia
  2. Nausea and vomiting
  3. Altered taste sensation
  4. Mucosal inflammation
  5. Dysphagia. Dysphagia, or difficulty in swallowing, may be relieved with a soft or pureed diet. Clients should take plenty of time to chew and swallow.
- Pain
- Fatigue
- Alopecia
- Odors
- Dyspnea
- Bowel dysfunctions
- Pathological fractures
- Ascites
- Sexual alterations

MEDICAL EMERGENCIES

Four complications with which nurses should become familiar are hypercalcemia, spinal cord compression, superior vena cava syndrome, and cardiac tamponade.

Hypercalcemia

Early symptoms of hypercalcemia, such as nausea, vomiting, constipation, and weakness, may be overlooked because these are common side effects of many cancer therapies. Later symptoms such as dehydration, renal failure, coma, and cardiac arrest may develop swiftly.

Hypercalcemia is treated aggressively with intravenous normal saline and furosemide (Lasix), which increase calcium excretion.

Spinal Cord Compression

Cancer of the lung, breast, and prostate carry the greatest risk of metastasizing to the spinal cord. The chief symptom of metastasis to the spinal cord is back pain. The discomfort is aggravated by lying down, coughing, or moving, and may be relieved by sitting upright.

Superior Vena Cava Syndrome

Superior vena cava syndrome is a collection of symptoms caused by an obstruction of the superior vena cava. Typically, clients experience dyspnea and swelling of the face and neck.

The client should be encouraged to limit activities and lie in Fowler's position. Respirations should be carefully monitored, and lower extremities should not be elevated, as doing so will increase venous return to an already engorged area.

Cardiac Tamponade

Cardiac tamponade is caused by the formation of pericardial fluid, which reduces cardiac output by compressing the heart. Common symptoms of cardiac tamponade include a rapid, weak pulse; distended neck veins during inspiration; ankle or sacral edema; pleural effusion; ascites; enlarged spleen; lethargy; and altered consciousness.

PSYCHOSOCIAL ALTERATIONS

The mere diagnosis of cancer invokes fear and misunderstanding. A myriad of emotions may surface initially. These may range from deep depression to denial and total refusal of treatment. Anxiety, sadness, and withdrawal are common.

Clients who seek information or share feelings tend to cope more effectively than do those who submit to treatment and procedures without asking questions or who use small talk to avoid discussing threatening issues.

NURSING CARE OF THE CLIENT: RESPIRATORY SYSTEM

ASSESSMENT

Note the client's color, level of consciousness, and emotional state. Observe respirations as to their rate, depth, quality, rhythm, and the effort required to breathe. Note symmetry of chest wall movement. Observe for use of accessory muscles to aid breathing. The position the client assumes provides information on respiratory status as individuals having trouble breathing often lean forward. Talbe 18-1 lists Respiratory Terms.

Assessment and Respiratory Assistive Devices

When caring for clients with respiratory assistive devices in place, the following must be assessed:

- Oxygen
  —Mode of delivery (e.g., nasal cannula, face mask)
  —Percentage of oxygen that is being delivered (e.g., 25%, 40%)
  —Flow rate of the oxygen (e.g., 2 liters per minute, 4 liters per minute)
  —Humidification provided and oxygen warmed

- Incentive Spirometer
  —Frequency of use
  —Volume achieved
  —Number of times client
  —reaches goal with each use

Auscultation

Assess breath sounds for duration, pitch, and intensity.

Adventitious Breath Sounds

Abnormal breath sounds are called adventitious breath sounds (see Table 18–2).

Pneumonia

Pneumonia is inflammation of the bronchioles and alveoli accompanied by consolidation, or solidification of exudate, in the lungs.

Medical–Surgical Management

Diet

The client with pneumonia is encouraged to drink fluids. Small, frequent, nutritionally balanced meals are preferred.

Table 18–1 RESPIRATORY TERMS

TERM	DEFINITION
Eupnea	Normal breathing
Apnea	Cessation of breathing, possibly temporary in nature
Dyspnea	Labored or difficult breathing, possibly normal if associated with exercise
Bradypnea	Abnormally slow breathing
Tachypnea	Abnormally rapid breathing
Orthopnea	Discomfort or difficulty with breathing in any but an upright sitting or standing position
Kussmaul's respirations	Abnormal respiratory pattern characterized by irregular periods of increased rate and depth of respiration; most often seen with diabetic ketoacidosis
Biot's respirations	Abnormal respiratory pattern characterized by irregular periods of apnea alternating with short periods of respiration of equal depth; most commonly seen with increased intracranial pressure
Cheyne-Stokes respirations	Abnormal respiratory pattern characterized by initially slow, shallow respirations that increase in rapidity and depth and then gradually decrease until respiration stops for 10 to 60 seconds; pattern then repeats itself in the same manner
Anoxia	Without oxygen
Hypoxia	Lack of adequate oxygen in inspired air such as occurs at high altitude
Hypoxemia	Insufficient amount of oxygen in the blood possibly due to respiratory, cardiovascular, or anemia-related disorders
Cyanosis	Bluish, grayish, or purplish discoloration of the skin due to abnormal amounts of reduced (oxygen-poor) hemoglobin in the blood; not always a reliable indicator of hypoxia
Acrocyanosis	Cyanosis of the fingertips and toes; often due to vasomotor disturbances associated with vasoconstriction
Circumoral cyanosis	Bluish discoloration encircling the mouth
Oxygen saturation	Amount of oxygen combined with hemoglobin

Assessment

Subjective Data

Onset, duration, and severity of cough; color, amount, and odor of sputum, if present; onset and duration of elevated temperature; presence or absence of night sweats.

Objective Data

Client's level of consciousness should be noted. Evidence of dyspnea, orthopnea, tachypnea, and cyanosis may be present.

Nursing Interventions

Nursing interventions for a client with pneumonia may include the following:

1. Obtain a sputum specimen for culture and sensitivity prior to initiating antibiotic therapy.
2. Encourage the client to breathe deeply and cough a minimum of every 2 hours.
3. Teach use of the incentive spirometer to encourage lung expansion.
4. Administer aerosol and nebulizer treatments as ordered.
5. Assess breath sounds and respiratory rate prior to and following respiratory procedures to evaluate their effectiveness.
6. Encourage fluids to liquefy thickened secretions.
7. For clients who are able, assist in sitting up or ambulating three to four times daily.
8. For the client who is on bed rest, turn every 2 hours.
9. Provide oral care several times a day.
10. Monitor pulse oximetry and/or ABGs.

Tuberculosis

Pulmonary tuberculosis (TB) is an infection of the lung tissue by *Mycobacterium tuberculosis*.

Medical–Surgical Management

Pharmacological
Active TB is treated with a combination of medications.

Nursing Interventions

Nursing interventions for a client with TB may include the following:

1. Assess the client's color, respiratory rate, and respiratory effort.
2. Auscultate the breath sounds.
3. Obtain sputum specimens for AFB; note the amount, color, and viscosity of the sputum.
4. Encourage fluids if not otherwise contraindicated.
5. Teach client and family about the basic pathophysiology of TB, how the infection is contracted, who is at risk of developing an infection, the signs and symptoms of TB infection, and complications that may arise.
6. Present information regarding the actions, side effects, and untoward effects of the drugs being administered.
7. Emphasize the necessity of long-term therapy to cure TB.
8. Inform the client and family that symptoms decrease and are often gone long before the organism is eliminated from the body.

Infection Control: Use of an N95 Particulate Respirator
- Follow facility's procedure for fit-testing
- Use the correct size mask
- Put on respirator before entering client's room and remove after leaving client's room
- Check that the seal between face and respirator is intact

Table 18–2 CHARACTERISTICS OF ADVENTITIOUS BREATH SOUNDS (ABNORMAL BREATH SOUNDS)

BREATH SOUND	RESPIRATORY PHASE	TIMING	DESCRIPTION
Fine crackle	Predominantly inspiration	Discontinuous	Dry, high-pitched crackling and popping of short duration: sounds like hair rolled between fingers when held near ears
Coarse crackle	Predominantly inspiration	Discontinuous	Moist, low-pitched crackling and gurgling of long duration
Sonorous wheeze	Predominantly expiration	Continuous	Low-pitched snoring
Sibilant wheeze	Predominantly expiration	Continuous	High-pitched and musical
Pleural friction rub	Inspiration and expiration	Continuous	Creaking, grating
Stridor	Predominantly inspiration	Continuous	Crowing

Adapted from Health Assessment & Physical Examination, *2nd ed., by M. E. Z. Estes, 2002, Albany, NY: Delmar. Copyright 2002 by Delmar. Adapted with permission.*

Pulmonary Embolism

Pulmonary embolism develops when a bloodborne substance lodges in a branch of a pulmonary artery and obstructs flow. A common source of pulmonary embolism is a deep vein thrombus.

Nursing Interventions

Nursing interventions for a client with pulmonary embolism may include the following:

1. Assess the client for indications of decreasing oxygenation.

CLEAR WITH COUGH	ETIOLOGY	CONDITIONS
Possibly	Air passing through moisture in small airways that suddenly reinflate	Chronic obstructive pulmonary disease (COPD), congestive heart failure (CHF), pneumonia, pulmonary fibrosis, atelectasis
Possibly	Air passing through moisture in large airways that suddenly reinflate	Pneumonia, pulmonary edema, bronchitis, atelectasis
Possibly	Narrowing of large airways or obstruction of bronchus	Asthma, bronchitis, airway edema, tumor, bronchiolar spasm, foreign body obstruction
Possibly	Narrowing of large airways or obstruction of bronchus	Asthma, chronic bronchitis, emphysema, tumor, foreign body obstruction
Never	Inflamed parietal and visceral pleura; can occasionally be felt on thoracic wall as two pieces of dry leather rubbing against each other	Pleurisy, tuberculosis, pulmonary infarction, pneumonia, lung abscess
Never	Partial obstruction of the larynx, trachea	Croup, foreign body obstruction, large airway tumor

2. Encourage deep breathing and coughing.
3. Provide supplemental oxygen to maintain oxygen saturation at greater than 95% or as ordered.
4. Administer subcutaneous heparin as ordered.
5. After anticoagulation is established, administer Coumadin as ordered.
6. Observe for side effects of anticoagulant therapy.

Pulmonary Edema

Acute pulmonary edema is a life-threatening condition characterized by a rapid shift of fluid from plasma into the pulmonary interstitial tissue and the alveoli.

Medical–Surgical Management

Arterial blood gases and pulse oximetry values are used to assess oxygenation.

Nursing Interventions

Nursing interventions for a client with pulmonary edema may include the following:

1. Place the client in high Fowler's or orthopneic position (sitting upright).
2. Continually assess oxygenation with ABG or pulse oximetry measurements and provide supplemental oxygen to maintain an oxygen saturation of 95% or greater or per physician's order.
3. Frequently assess respiratory rate, breath sounds, apical heart rate, and blood pressure. Administer respiratory treatments as ordered.
4. Assist the client with activities to reduce the workload on the heart and lungs, and alternate periods of activity with periods of rest to prevent client fatigue.
5. Administer medications as ordered and evaluate the effectiveness of each.
6. Monitor lab reports for electrolyte values.
7. Weigh client daily.
8. Monitor I&O.

9. Frequently assess the client for peripheral edema.

Adult Respiratory Distress Syndrome

Adult respiratory distress syndrome (ARDS) is a life-threatening condition characterized by severe dyspnea, hypoxemia, and diffuse pulmonary edema.

Nursing Interventions

Nursing interventions for a client with ARDS may include the following:

1. Provide adequate oxygenation and ventilation as ordered.
2. Monitor ABGs and pulse oximetry to evaluate oxygenation and acid–base balance.
3. Assess the client's respiratory rate and effort and auscultate the lungs frequently.
4. Suction the respiratory tract as necessary to remove excess secretions.

Emphysema

Emphysema is a complex and destructive lung disease wherein air accumulates in the tissues of the lungs. The airways become fibrotic and lose their elasticity, resulting in narrower lumens. Airflow is impeded as it leaves the lungs (i.e., during expiration). The alveoli distal to these airways become overdistended with trapped air. Rupture of the alveolar wall may occur. The alveolar capillary membrane is destroyed, resulting in a loss of available area for gas exchange.

Nursing Interventions

Nursing interventions for a client with emphysema may include the following:

1. Assess the client's level of consciousness and mental status.
2. Frequently evaluate the client's respiratory rate, respiratory effort, and color.
3. Evaluate oxygenation with ABG and/or pulse oximetry measurement.
4. Assess the effect of activity on oxygenation, particularly when activity is being increased.
5. Assess the client's vital signs: Heart rate and temperature elevations may indicate infection. An elevated pulse can also indicate hypoxia.
6. Assist the client in assuming the position that offers the most comfort and that most aids respiratory effort.
7. Assist the client with ADL and hygiene needs.
8. Administer medications and respiratory treatments prior to meals to aid in breathing.

Bronchiectasis

Bronchiectasis is chronic dilation of the bronchi.

Pneumothorax/ Hemothorax

Pneumothorax is an accumulated air or gas in the pleural space. The lung tissue underlying the pneumothorax is compressed and thus unable to fully expand. If the pneumothorax is large enough, the underlying lung tissue collapses as a result of the compression.

If hypoxia results from compromised breathing, activity restrictions are necessary. After the client is adequately oxygenated and stable, activity is encouraged to promote expansion of the lungs.

Nursing Interventions

Nursing interventions for a client with a pneumothorax may include the following:

1. Monitor the amount and character of drainage from the chest tube.
2. Note any drainage from the chest tube as output.
3. Observe for the presence of bubbling in the water seal chamber, which is indicative of an air leak. Assess the connections and chest tube to determine whether leaks are present. If no air leaks are present, notify the physician as to the possibility of an air leak within the client's lungs.
4. Encourage the client to cough and deep breathe to prevent further respiratory complications.

Lung Cancer

Malignant tumors (carcinomas) of the lung may originate within the lung itself or may result from metastasis from other tumor sites (e.g., breast, colon, or kidney).

Nursing Interventions

Nursing interventions for a client with lung cancer may include the following:

1. Assess pain as to its location, character, duration, and severity.
2. Note the color, amount, consistency, and odor of sputum.
3. Administer pain medication as ordered.
4. Monitor for respiratory depression.

Laryngeal Cancer

Cancer of the larynx.

Daily Stoma Care

After the stoma has healed:

- Use warm water to clean around the stoma.
- Do not use tissues, linty cotton, or soap for cleansing.
- Wear a bib or dressing over the stoma to filter and warm incoming air.
- Humidify home, especially in winter.
- Do not swim or splash water in the stoma when showering or bathing.

- Notify the physician if any signs of respiratory infection develop, such as fever, cough, yellow or green mucus, or redness around the stoma.

Nursing Interventions

Nursing interventions for a client with laryngeal cancer may include the following:

1. Before surgery, establish a means of communication to be used afterwards. If available, a manual or computer word/picture board works well.
2. Keep call light by client's bed.
3. Avoid mouthing communications, as this is frustrating to the client and is time consuming.
4. As possible, ask questions that require only a "yes" or "no" answer.
5. Refer the client to the local support group (Lost Chord Club) or the American Cancer Society.
6. Suction frequently following surgery to remove static secretions.
7. Provide routine tracheostomy care.
8. Teach client stoma care and protection.

NURSING CARE OF THE CLIENT: CARDIOVASCULAR SYSTEM

CHAPTER 1

ASSESSMENT

Assessment includes clients' self-report of symptoms as well as physical findings and confirming lab data.

Subjective Data

Listen carefully to explanations of the client's activity level or limitations in activity. Ask about sleeping habits to evaluate the client's ability to sleep, i.e., the need for the trunk of the body to be supported with pillows when sleeping, or the need to sleep in a chair.

It is important to ascertain the onset of the pain, situation occurring at the onset of pain, location and radiation of pain, severity of chest pain, duration, past episodes of chest pain, and methods used to alleviate pain.

Objective Data

Carefully assess the skin, neck veins, respirations, heart sounds, abdomen, and extremities. Check the peripheral pulses. Pulse amplitude can be rated on a scale of 0 to 4: 0 (absent), 1+ (diminished but palpable), 2+ (normal), 3+ (full, increased), and 4+ (bounding).

Note if the feet, ankles, or legs are edematous. Edema can be rated on a scale of 1 to 4: 1+ (barely visible), 2+ (obviously present), 3+ (able to indent, but rebounds when finger removed), 4+ (indentation remains when finger removed).

Observe for stasis dermatitis, an inflammation of the skin due to decreased circulation.

Dysrhythmias

A dysrhythmia is an irregularity in the rate, rhythm, or conduction of the electrical system of the heart.

BRADYCARDIA

Sinus bradycardia is a heart rate of 60 beats/minute or less.

TACHYCARDIA

Tachycardia is a sinus rhythm with a heart rate ranging from 100 to 150 beats/minute.

ATRIAL DYSRHYTHMIAS

Common causes for atrial dysrhythmias are myocardial infarction, congestive heart failure, electrolyte imbalances, emotional stress, and drugs.

Premature Atrial Contractions

A premature atrial contraction (PAC) is an ectopic impulse not originating in the sinoatrial node, but rather in the atrial tissue.

Atrial Tachycardia

Atrial tachycardia is an ectopic impulse that causes the atria to contract at the rate of 140 to 250 beats/minute.

Paroxysmal Supraventricular Tachycardia

Paroxysmal supraventricular tachycardia (PSVT) is a rapid atrial beat accompanied by an abnormal conduction in the AV node.

Atrial Flutter

Atrial flutter, a rapid contraction of the atria, yields a heart rate of 250 to 350 beats/minute (Figure 19-1).

Atrial Fibrillation

Atrial fibrillation is an erratic electrical activity of the atria, resulting in a rate of 350 to 600 beats/minute (Figure 19-1).

VENTRICULAR DYSRHYTHMIAS

Ventricular dysrhythmias are more life threatening than atrial dysrhythmias. They must be treated promptly.

Premature Ventricular Contractions

Premature ventricular contractions (PVCs) arise from ectopic beats in the ventricles and can easily be identified on the EKG because of the wide, bizarre QRS complexes. There are no P waves preceding the QRS complex (Figure 19-3).

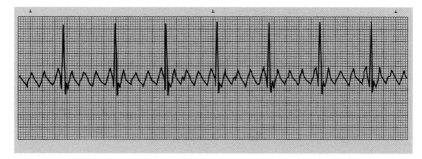

Figure 19-1 Atrial Flutter

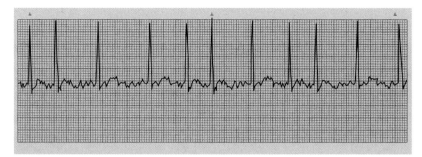

Figure 19-2 Atrial Fibrillation

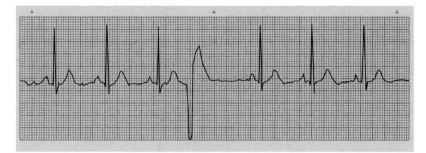

Figure 19-3 Premature Ventricular Contractions

Ventricular Tachycardia

The ventricular rate is 100 beats/minute and may go as high as 140 to 240 beats/minute. Underlying conditions in which VT occurs are cardiomyopathy, hypoxemia, digitalis toxicity, and electrolyte imbalance.

Ventricular Fibrillation

VF is a disorganized, chaotic quivering of the ventricles (Figure 19-4).

Ventricular Asystole

Ventricular asystole is represented only by a P wave or by a straight line on the EKG. The ventricles are not contracting and the client is in cardiac arrest (Figure 19-5).

ATRIOVENTRICULAR BLOCKS

First Degree AV Block

In first degree block the impulse is delayed in traveling through the AV node (Figure 19-6).

Second Degree AV Block

In second degree block some of the impulses pass through the AV

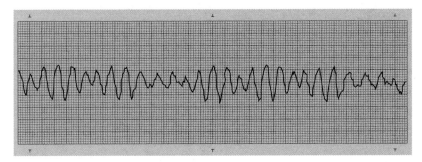

Figure 19-4 Ventricular Fibrillation

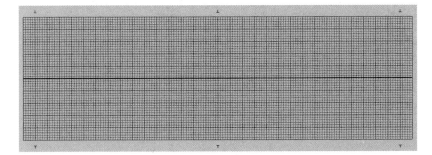

Figure 19-5 Asystole

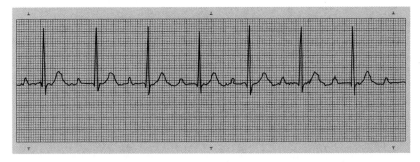

Figure 19-6 First Degree AV Block

node to the ventricles and others are blocked (Figure 19-7).

Type I AV block is usually caused by a drug toxicity and is treated by withholding the drug. Type I may also occur with an acute inferior wall myocardial infarction. Type II is more serious than type I and indicates a blockage in the conduction in the bundle of His or the bundle branches (compare Figure 19-6 and Figure 19-7).

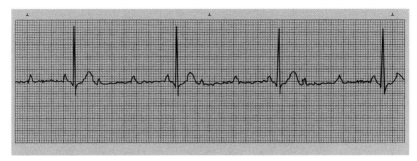

Figure 19-7 Second Degree AV block: Mobitz's Type II

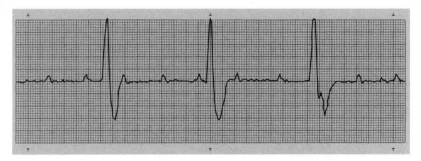

Figure 19-8 Third Degree AV Block

Third Degree AV Block

Third degree heart block is when no impulses are able to pass from the atria through the AV node to the ventricles (Figure 19-8).

Mitral Valve Prolapse

Mitral insufficiency can lead to mitral valve prolapse in which the valve leaflets, chordae tendineae, and papillary muscle become damaged. The valve leaflets flip back into the left atrium when the left ventricle contracts.

Nursing Interventions

Nursing interventions for a client with cardiac valvular disorders may include the following:

1. Administer oxygen as needed.
2. Help the client balance activities with rest periods. The pulse should return to the baseline within 10 minutes of activity; if not, activity has been excessive.
3. Discourage smoking and refer clients to support groups to assist them to stop smoking.

Refer to Table 19-1 for other valve problems.

Table 19–1 MITRAL AND AORTIC VALVE STENOSIS AND INSUFFICIENCY

VALVE CONDITION	DEFINITION	SYMPTOMS
Mitral stenosis	The diseased valve becomes narrowed and the leaflets thickened, preventing blood from freely flowing from the left atrium into the left ventricle.	Gradual onset of symptoms: exertional dyspnea, fatigue, orthopnea, paroxysmal nocturnal dyspnea, murmur. **Later symptoms:** peripheral edema, atrial fibrillation, jugular venous distention, hepatomegaly, abdominal distention, hypotension, thrombus from blood pooling in the left atrium.
Mitral Insufficiency	The valve leaflets become hard and do not close completely. Blood backs up in both the left atria and ventricle, causing both chambers to hypertrophy.	Gradual onset of symptoms: exertional dyspnea, palpitations, fatigue, atrial fibrillation, loud murmur and gallop.
Aortic Stenosis	The valve cusps become hard and calcify due to rheumatic fever, syphilis, a congenital anomaly, or the aging process.	Syncope, exertional dyspnea, arrhythmias, angina, murmur, and gallop; sudden death may occur. **Later symptoms as the disease progresses:** paroxysmal atrial tachycardia, orthopnea.
Aortic Insufficiency	The valve cusps become so hardened they do not close completely. The blood no longer flows through the aorta but backs up into the left ventricle.	Palpitations, chest pain, exertional dyspnea, nocturnal angina, dizziness, fatigue, decreased activity, intolerance, paroxysmal nocturnal dyspnea, visible pulsation of the neck veins, murmur, lung congestion.

DIAGNOSTIC FINDINGS	MEDICAL–SURGICAL MANAGEMENT	NURSING INTERVENTIONS
Chest x-ray: hypertrophy and enlargement of left atrium and right ventricle. **EKG:** atrial fibrillation. **Echocardiogram:** fusion of valve leaflets, enlarged left atrium, decreased blood flow through valve.	**Medical management:** diuretics, digitalis, anticoagulants, antidysrhythmics,prophylactic antibiotics for invasive procedures, low-sodium diet, semi-Fowler's position, activity restrictions as needed. **Surgical management:** commissurotomy, percutaneous balloon mitral valvuloplasty, mitral valve replacement.	Encourage rest periods, administer oxygen, elevate head of bed, reposition frequently to decrease pressure points, elevate legs, low-sodium diet, monitor for signs of right and left-sided heart failure, teach stress reduction techniques, daily weight.
Chest x-ray: hypertrophy and enlargement of left atrium and left ventricle. **EKG:** atrial fibrillation.	**Medical management:** same as mitral stenosis. **Surgical management:** valvuloplasty, mitral valve replacement.	Same as mitral stenosis. Teach exercise modification.
Chest x-ray: enlargement of left ventricle, calcification of aortic valve. **EKG:** hypertrophy of left ventricle inverted T wave. **Echocardiogram:** fusion of valve leaflets, regurgitation.	**Medical management:** same as mitral stenosis. **Surgical management:** percutaneous balloon aortic valvuloplasty, aortic valve replacement.	Same as mitral stenosis.
Chest x-ray: hypertrophy and enlargement of left ventricle.	**Medical management:** same as mitral stenosis. **Surgical management:** aortic valve replacement.	Same as mitral stenosis. Teach exercise modification.

Arteriosclerosis

Arteriosclerosis is a narrowing and hardening of arteries.

Angina Pectoris

Myocardial ischemia is a temporary inadequate blood and oxygen supply to the myocardial tissues. When this temporary condition occurs, the person experiences chest pain or angina pectoris.

Myocardial Infarction

A myocardial infarction is caused by an obstruction in a coronary artery resulting in necrosis (death) to the tissues supplied by the artery.

Nursing Interventions

Nursing interventions for a client with myocardial infarction may include the following:

1. Maintain bed rest with head of bed elevated 30° until the condition is stabilized.
2. Administer oxygen per mask or nasal cannula at 2 to 4 liters per minute.
3. If beta-blockers are administered, monitor closely for a drop in heart rate and blood pressure.
4. Constantly monitor the client for dysrhythmias. Place a rhythm strip on the chart at least once a shift.
5. Monitor I&O.
6. Administer analgesic, usually morphine, as ordered.

Congestive Heart Failure

Congestive heart failure develops when the heart is no longer capable of meeting the oxygen needs of the body. The muscle of the left ventricle hypertrophies (increases in muscle mass) and often the ventricular chamber enlarges in an attempt to meet the oxygen needs of the body.

Both the right and left ventricles can fail separately resulting in two types of heart failure: right-sided heart failure and left-sided heart failure. Heart failure usually begins on the left side.

Nursing Interventions

Nursing interventions for a client with congestive heart failure may include the following:

1. Take an apical pulse on all cardiac clients, especially checking the rate and rhythm.
2. Monitor the client's heart rate and rhythm by telemetry.
3. Closely monitor the electrolytes, especially the potassium level, as diuretics can deplete the potassium level.
4. Take the apical pulse before giving a digitalis preparation. If the heart rate is below 60, withhold the medication and notify the physician. In some institutions the heart rate can drop to 50 before the physician is notified if the client is taking a calcium channel blocker or beta-blocker along with digitalis.

5. Provide oxygen by mask or nasal cannula at 2 to 6 liters/minute.
6. Elevate the head of the bed to a semi-Fowler's or Fowler's position.
7. Apply a pulse oximeter and monitor the oxygenation status. If the pulse oximeter is ≤90%, notify the physician.
8. Encourage elevation of the client's legs, not letting them hang in a dependent position.
9. Monitor daily fluids by obtaining an accurate intake and output.
10. Take a daily weight at the same time each day, on the same scales, and with the client wearing the same type of clothing.

Aneurysm

An aneurysm is a localized dilation occurring in a weakened section of an artery's medial layer.

Assessment

After a surgical aneurysm repair, the extremities are assessed for color, warmth, peripheral pulses, and sensation.

Nursing Interventions

Nursing interventions for a client with an aneurysm may include the following:

1. Monitor for symptoms of an occluded vessel (pain, paleness, cyanosis, and coldness).
2. Monitor the temperature, color, and fullness of the peripheral pulses in both extremities and compare them to the preoperative pulses.
3. Measure hourly output to make sure the client has at least 25 to 30 cc of urine per hour.
4. Monitor vital signs closely for signs of hemorrhage.
5. Check the operative site frequently to make sure the dressing is dry. Turn the client to make sure blood is not pooling under the client's body. Monitor for other signs of hemorrhaging.
6. Measure the abdomen for increasing abdominal girth indicating internal bleeding. If the client has low back pain, there may be hemorrhaging in the retroperitoneal space. Other symptoms of hemorrhage are lightheadedness, dizziness, and tachycardia
7. Check for adequate functioning and drainage of the NG tube to decrease pressure on the aneurysm repair site and incision.

Hypertension

Hypertension (HTN), also known as high blood pressure, is defined as an elevated arterial blood pressure. A systolic blood pressure above 140 or a diastolic blood pressure above 90 is indicative of hypertension.

Often the hypertensive client may not be experiencing any symptoms and does not see the importance of caring effectively for this condition.

Medical–Surgical Management

The first step is to encourage the client to try some diet and lifestyle changes. These include losing weight if the client is more than 15% over the optimum weight; limiting sodium, saturated fat, cholesterol, and alcohol intake; exercising on a regular basis; stopping the use of nicotine; and maintaining an adequate intake of calcium, magnesium, and potassium.

Nursing Interventions

Nursing interventions for a client with hypertension may include the following:

1. Make referrals to the appropriate personnel to teach the client lifestyle changes. These may include a dietitian, smoking cessation clinic, fitness center, or stress management seminars.
2. Explain the pathophysiology, risk factors, lifestyle changes, medication actions and side effects, and complications of hypertension.
3. Regularly inquire about the client's satisfaction in regard to the prescribed regimen of diet, exercise, and prescribed medications.
4. If the client cannot afford needed medications, refer the client to financial assistance programs.
5. Encourage the client to become an active participant in the treatment as this will give the client a sense of control over the condition.
6. Encourage the client to record BP readings, weekly weight, exercise activities, and dietary intake as a way of giving a sense of control and encouraging compliance.
7. Give basic dietary instructions or make a referral to a dietician.
8. Weigh the client at scheduled appointments.
9. Since diuretics and antihypertensive medications may cause impotence, discuss this effect in an open and candid manner, so the client and spouse will be open to discuss difficulties in this area.

NURSING CARE OF THE CLIENT: HEMATOLOGIC AND LYMPHATIC SYSTEMS

ASSESSMENT

Subjective Data

Inquire about the client's occupation and hobbies as there may be exposure to radiation or chemicals. Past military experience is also important, as some military personnel have been exposed to toxic chemicals. Obtain medication history from the client, including prescription and over-the-counter medications. Note recent or recurring infections, night sweats, palpitations, bleeding problems, previous blood transfusions and any complications.

Assess neurological functioning by asking if the client has experienced any cognitive or mental difficulties or numbness and tingling of the extremities. A headache may be indicative of a low erythrocyte count or intracranial bleeding. Note hearing or vision difficulties.

Ask the client about past surgeries and any complications from surgeries. Inquire about alcohol use. Ask the client about the presence of blood in the stool or urine and any anorexia, nausea, vomiting, oral dis-

comfort, or problems with taste perception. Inquire if the client has difficulty accomplishing ADLs because of decreased energy.

Objective Data

Palpate the lymph nodes in the neck, axillae, and groin; normal findings include small (0.5–1.0 cm) nodes that are freely movable, firm, and nontender.

Inspect the skin and extremities for petechiae, bruises, lesions, and brittle nails. Check urine and stool for blood. Document dyspnea, an enlarged abdomen, or swollen joints.

Iron Deficiency Anemia

Iron deficiency anemia occurs when the body does not have enough iron to synthesize functional Hgb. This condition may be due to decreased dietary intake, decreased iron absorption from the gastrointestinal tract, chronic intestinal or uterine blood loss, or an increased bodily need for iron such as during growth periods or pregnancy.

Hypoplastic (Aplastic) Anemia

The client with aplastic anemia has pancytopenia, a drop in the number of red blood cells, white blood cells, and platelets because the bone marrow decreases or stops functioning.

Pernicious Anemia

Pernicious anemia is an autoimmune disease resulting from a lack of protein intrinsic factor necessary for the absorption of vitamin B_{12}.

Acquired Hemolytic Anemia

In hemolytic anemias, there is a premature destruction of RBCs.

Sickle Cell Anemia

This genetic disorder has abnormal hemoglobin S rather than hemoglobin A in the RBCs.

Nursing Interventions

Nursing interventions for a client with decreased erythrocytes and hemoglobin may include the following:

1. Teach the cause of the particular type of anemia and, if possible, ways to avoid the occurrence of that anemia in the future.
2. For iron deficiency anemia, teach the importance of taking iron and increasing iron in the diet.
3. Instruct clients with pernicious anemia to obtain a vitamin B_{12} injection at regularly scheduled times.

4. Teach clients with hemolytic anemias the significance of following the prescribed regimens.
5. Teach clients with sickle cell anemia to have adequate fluid intake as dehydration causes a sickle cell crisis.
6. Monitor Hgb, Hct, RBCs, ABGs, and electrolytes.
7. Monitor vital signs and mental alertness.
8. Monitor for symptoms of obstructed vessels such as pain, leg ulcerations, abdominal tenderness, dyspnea, confusion, and blurred vision.
9. Monitor the client closely after blood transfusions for possible reactions such as chills, fever, dyspnea, pruritus, wheezing, and pain in the lumbar region.

Polycythemia

Polycythemia is a disease in which there is an increased production of red blood cells. Usually the numbers of white blood cells and platelets are also increased. The increased production of cells increases the blood volume and viscosity and decreases the ability of the blood to circulate freely.

Nursing Interventions

Nursing interventions for a client with polycythemia may include the following:

1. Encourage the client to drink 3 L of water daily.
2. Teach client to report headache, chest pain, dyspnea, or redness,

swelling, or tenderness in the arms or legs to the physician or nurse practitioner immediately.

3. Encourage the client to change positions slowly to prevent dizziness.

WHITE BLOOD CELL DISORDERS

Leukemia

Leukemia is a malignancy of blood-forming tissues in which the bone marrow produces increased numbers of immature white blood cells that are incapable of protecting the body from infections. WBCs crowd out the other cells in the bone marrow, causing a decreased production of RBCs and platelets.

Leukemia has two classifications: acute and chronic. The acute leukemias are subclassified into acute myelocytic leukemia (AML) and acute lymphocytic leukemia (ALL). Chronic leukemias are subclassified into chronic myelocytic leukemia (CML) and chronic lymphocytic leukemia (CLL).

Nursing Interventions

Nursing interventions for a client with leukemia may include the following:

1. Follow good handwashing techniques.
2. Provide frequent oral care with a soft toothbrush and nonirritating mouthwash to prevent open sores and stomatitis.

3. Wash the perianal area after each bowel movement to decrease bacterial contamination and prevent rectal fissures.
4. Avoid taking a rectal temperature and giving suppositories.
5. Report any temperature over 100°F to the physician.
6. Closely monitor respiration rate and breath sounds as the client is prone to respiratory infections.
7. Frequently observe the client for signs of bleeding such as epistaxis, gingival bleeding, petechiae, ecchymoses, hematemesis, enlarged abdomen, hematuria, melena, and confusion, which can occur from intracranial hemorrhage.
8. If a catheter is needed, lubricate it well to avoid trauma to the mucosal lining of the urethra.
9. Encourage the client to voice concerns and fears related to having leukemia.

Agranulocytosis

Agranulocytosis is a severely reduced number of granulocytes (basophils, eosinophils, and neutrophils).

Nursing Interventions

Nursing interventions for a client with agranulocytosis may include the following:

1. Thoroughly wash hands before caring for the client.
   Screen all persons for signs of infection before allowing them near the client.
2. Monitor vital signs for signs of infection.

Use strict asepsis for all procedures.

3. Encourage the client to drink an adequate amount of fluids.

Thrombocytopenia

Thrombocytopenia is a decrease in the number of platelets in the blood.

Nursing Interventions

Nursing interventions for a client with thrombocytopenia may include the following:

1. Assess client's pain on 0 (least) to 10 (most) pain scale.
2. Monitor client's vital signs and neurological and mental status.
3. Assess client's skin and excretions for signs of bleeding.

LYMPH DISORDERS

Hodgkin's Disease

Hodgkin's disease is a rare lymphoma that usually arises as a painless swelling in a lymph node. The diagnosis is confirmed when Reed-Sternberg cells are biopsied from the swollen lymph node.

Non-Hodgkin's Lymphoma

NHL originates from the B lymphocytes and the T lymphocytes. NHL arising from the B lymphocyte occurs in the older adult population; NHL arising from the T lymphocytes manifests in malignant skin diseases such as mycosis fungoides or Sezary syndrome.

Nursing Interventions

Nursing interventions for a client with Hodgkin's disease or non-Hodgkin's disease may include the following:

1. Encourage the client to take frequent deep breaths to expand the lungs and prevent infection.
2. Provide cool sponge baths or oral medication to relieve pruritus.
3. Encourage the client to report symptoms of dyspnea, sore throat, and burning or frequency of urination.
4. Encourage an adequate intake of fluids to prevent constipation and renal stones.

PLASMA CELL DISORDER

Multiple Myeloma

Plasma cells become malignant, crowd out normal cell production, destroy normal bone tissue, and thereby cause pain.

Nursing Interventions

Nursing interventions for a client with multiple myeloma may include the following:

1. Assess the client's pain level with pain scale.

2. Reposition the client using a lift sheet.
3. Teach the client and family proper handwashing.
4. Encourage the client to drink 3–4 L of fluids per day.
5. Monitor for symptoms of hypercalcemia and notify physician if symptoms occur.

NURSING CARE OF THE CLIENT: INTEGUMENTARY SYSTEM

ASSESSMENT

Inspection and palpation are the two assessment techniques used when examining the skin. Table 21–1 outlines the seven parameters of examination with normal and abnormal findings.

Wound Drainage

Serous exudate is watery in appearance and has a low protein level. This type of exudate is seen with mild inflammation resulting in minimal capillary permeability changes and minimal protein molecule escape (e.g., seen in blister formation after a burn).

Purulent exudate is pus. Purulent exudates may vary in color (e.g., yellow, green, brown) depending on the causative organism.

Hemorrhagic exudate reflects whether the bleeding is fresh or old (bright red versus dark red).

Serosanguineous exudate is clear with some blood tinge and is seen with surgical incisions.

Location

Assessment begins with a description of the anatomical location of the wound, for example, "5-inch suture line on the right lower quadrant of the abdomen."

Size

The length (head to toe), width (side to side), and depth of a wound are measured in centimeters. If tunneling is noted, the location and depth are documented.

General Appearance and Drainage

Describe the color of the wound and surrounding area.

Pain

Notify the physician of any pain or tenderness at the wound site.

Burns

Figure 21-1 depicts the various layers of skin involved in burn injuries.

Table 21-1 SKIN ASSESSMENT PARAMETERS

PARAMETER	NORMAL	ABNORMAL
Integrity	Skin intact; no diseased or injured tissue.	Broken skin; open areas such as fissures, ulcers, excoriations. Rash or lesions such as papules, nodules, vesicles, pustules, wheals, scales.
Color	Varies with skin type and race: pink, tanned, olive, brown.	Pallor—pale skin, especially in face, conjunctiva, nail beds, and oral mucous membranes. Cyanosis—bluish discoloration noticed in lips, earlobes, and nail beds. Jaundice—a yellowing of the skin, mucous membranes, and sclera. Erythema—reddish hue to the skin as in sunburn and inflammation.
Temperature and moisture	Usually warm and dry, depending on environmental temperature.	Cool, cold, moist, clammy, or warmer than normal.
Texture	Smooth, soft. Thickness varies in different areas.	Loose, wrinkled, rough, thickened, thin, oily, flaking, scaling.
Turgor and mobility	An assessment of skin hydration. Normally skin moves freely. A pinched fold of skin returns immediately to normal position.	Taut with edema; slack with dehydration. Rigid in some diseases such as scleroderma.
Sensation	Distinguishes hot and cold, sharp and dull.	Numbness, tingling, insensitive to pressure and sharp objects.
Vascularity	Clear; no discoloration.	Telangiectasia (permanent dilation of groups of superficial capillaries and venules); Petechiae (pinpoint hemorrhagic spots); Ecchymosis (large, irregular, hemorrhagic areas).

Nursing Interventions

Nursing interventions for a client with a burn injury may include the following:

1. Administer intravenous fluids at the ordered rate.

2. Monitor for signs and symptoms of fluid overload such as shortness of breath, crackles auscultated in lung bases, changes in heart rate and/or heart sounds, changes in blood pressure, increased anxiety, or changes in mental status.

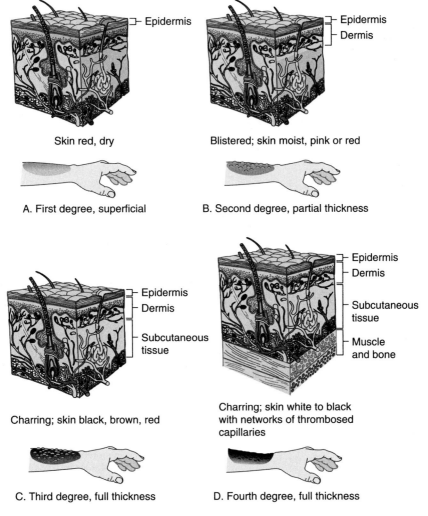

Skin red, dry

A. First degree, superficial

Blistered; skin moist, pink or red

B. Second degree, partial thickness

Charring; skin black, brown, red

C. Third degree, full thickness

Charring; skin white to black with networks of thrombosed capillaries

D. Fourth degree, full thickness

Figure 21-1 Skin Layers Involved in Burn Injuries: A. First-degree burn; B. Second-degree burn; C. Third-degree burn; D. Fourth-degree burn

3. Measure urine output hourly, report outputs below 30 mL to the physician.
4. When the client can tolerate oral fluids, set a fluid intake goal for each shift (e.g., 1,200 mL during the day; 800 mL during the evening; 500 mL during the night).
5. Monitor for signs and symptoms of electrolyte imbalances such as increased muscle weakness,

muscle cramps, cardiac arrhythmias, fatigue, nausea, dizziness.

During the stabilization and recovery period following a burn, the nursing interventions may include the following:

1. Monitor wound daily for signs of infection: redness, swelling, purulent drainage, pain.
2. Assess for signs of systemic infections.
3. Observe for increased pulse and respirations, decreased blood pressure, and fever.

Other nursing interventions common to most clients with burns include the following:

1. Assess for pain every 2 to 4 hours by asking client to rate pain level on a scale of 0 to 10.
2. Administer pain medications as ordered, especially prior to wound care or exercise and mobilization activities.
3. Perform passive ROM exercises 4 times a day by supporting the limb above and below the joint and performing exercises slowly and smoothly.
4. Use splints as ordered by the physician to keep hands, wrists, feet, and ankles in natural alignment and explain the reason for these activities to the client.
5. Provide time for the client to express feelings (fear, anger, frustration, regret, and depression are commonly expressed by clients with burns) and practice active listening.

NEOPLASMS: MALIGNANT

Basal Cell Carcinoma

Basal cell carcinoma, the most frequent type of skin cancer, arises from the epidermis.

Squamous Cell Carcinoma

Squamous cell carcinoma appears as a nodular lesion in the epidermis.

Malignant Melanoma

Malignant melanoma is the most serious of the three types of skin cancers and may begin in a preexisting mole (nevus). These moles have an irregular shape, are larger than 6 mm in diameter, and do not have a uniform color. Malignant melanoma can metastasize to every organ in the body through the bloodstream and lymphatic system.

Mycosis Fungoides

Mycosis fungoides (cutaneous T-cell lymphoma) is a malignant disease involving T-helper cells that have both skin manifestations and multiple organ system manifestations. In the early stages it resembles psoriasis or seborrheic dermatitis. Later, fissures and skin ulcers develop. The disease is ultimately fatal because of the involvement of vital organ systems.

Ulcers

The two most common types of ulcers of the skin are stasis ulcers and pressure ulcers.

Stasis Ulcers

The skin changes in texture, turgor, and color; develops a brownish discoloration; subcutaneous tissue atrophies; and the texture loses its usual resiliency and feels hard to the touch.

Nursing Interventions

Nursing interventions for a client with a stasis ulcer may include the following:

1. Encourage the client to elevate legs while sitting or when in bed.
2. Advise the client to avoid standing for more than a few minutes at a time.
3. Advise client to wear elastic stockings when walking and that new stockings should be purchased every few months because continual wear and laundering tend to decrease the elasticity of the stockings.
4. Instruct not to wear garters, tight girdles, or sit with legs crossed.
5. Assess the ulcer daily for signs of healing.
6. Review diet with the client and instruct in food choices as needed. Encourage foods high in iron such as fortified cereal, lean meats, whole grains, and leafy green vegetables.

Pressure Ulcers

Pressure ulcers are localized areas of tissue necrosis that tend to develop when soft tissue is compressed between a bony prominence and an external surface such as a mattress or chair seat for a prolonged period of time.

Staging of pressure ulcers:

- Stage I: Nonblanchable erythema of intact skin; the heralding lesion of skin ulceration.
- Stage II: The ulcer is superficial and presents clinically as an abrasion, blister, or shallow crater.
- Stage III: The ulcer presents clinically as a deep crater with or without undermining of adjacent tissue.
- Stage IV: Undermining and sinus tracts may also be associated with stage IV pressure ulcers.

Nursing Interventions

Nursing interventions for a client at risk for pressure ulcers or who has a pressure ulcer may include the following:

1. Provide daily bath and skin care as needed for incontinence of urine or stool.
2. Use moisturizing lotion and minimize exposure to cold and low humidity.
3. Avoid massage over bony prominences.
4. Encourage adequate fluid intake and a well-balanced diet, including 2 half-cup servings of orange juice or other juice high in vitamin C and 6 ounces of a high-protein drink.

5. Turn and reposition client at least every 2 hours.
6. Use the 30° lateral position to avoid pressure on the sacrum and trochanters.
7. Use pressure-reducing surfaces.
8. Assess skin daily, identifying the stage of pressure ulcer development (size, color, odor, and exudate).

NURSING CARE OF THE CLIENT: IMMUNE SYSTEM

ASSESSMENT

The skin and mucous membranes are evaluated for urticaria, inflammation, or bleeding. Superficial head, neck, supraclavicular, axilla, and inguinal lymph nodes are inspected and palpated for redness, tenderness, or swelling. Evaluate joints for possible tenderness, swelling, or limited range of motion. Assess changes in the rate and rhythm of respirations, presence of a cough, or abnormal lung sounds. Assess cardiovascular status, including rate, rhythm, arrhythmias, and peripheral vascular circulation. Assess for enlarged liver or spleen and gastrointestinal conditions, such as nausea, vomiting, or diarrhea.

Anaphylactic Reaction

Anaphylaxis is a type I systemic reaction to allergens and is the most serious type of allergic reaction. Symptoms develop suddenly and can progress to severe levels within minutes.

Nursing Interventions

Nursing interventions for clients with anaphylaxis may include the following:

1. Monitor vital signs frequently.
2. Place client in modified Trendelenburg position for hypotension.
3. Administer IV fluids and medications as ordered.
4. Maintain patent airway.
5. Administer oxygen and medications as ordered.
6. Advise client to provide the name of the causative agent and a description of reaction experienced when asked about allergies.

Transfusion Reactions

There are 5 types of transfusion reactions: febrile nonhemolytic, allergic urticarial, delayed hemolytic, acute hemolytic, and anaphylactic. Febrile nonhemolytic reactions are the result of an antibody-antigen reaction to WBCs. Clients who have allergic urticarial reactions develop a skin rash during or within 1 hour following the transfusion. A delayed hemolytic reaction may occur days to weeks following the transfusion. The client's hemoglobin level falls. An acute hemolytic reaction is potentially a life-threatening situation. Symptoms resulting from the incompatibility of ABO groups usually occur during the first 15 minutes of administration, but can develop anytime during the transfusion. Clients complain of chills, nausea, and back pain. Fever, drop in blood pressure (hypotension), vomiting, hematuria, or oliguria may be observed. As the condition progresses, chest pain, dyspnea, anuria, and shock develop. Anaphylactic reactions, although rare, are also life-threatening. Symptoms of acute gastrointestinal malfunctioning and cardiovascular and respiratory collapse develop moments after the transfusion has started.

Nursing Interventions

A nursing intervention for clients with transfusion reactions may be:

1. Follow protocol for blood products and administration.
2. Check client's identification and blood product with another nurse.
3. If a reaction occurs, stop transfusion immediately, then call the physician.
4. Administer medications as ordered.
5. Send blood tubing and a urine specimen to the lab for analysis.
6. Monitor and document client's condition.
7. Teach client who has a blood transfusion reaction to inform health care providers whenever questioned about allergies.

AUTOIMMUNE DISEASES

Rheumatoid Arthritis

Rheumatoid arthritis (RA) is a chronic, systemic autoimmune disease characterized by joint stiffness.

Nursing Interventions

Nursing interventions for clients with rheumatoid arthritis may include the following:

1. Teach client use of assistive devices, such as handrests, tools to pick up objects, or three-legged canes, as needed.
2. Assist client to use handrails in tub, shower, and toilet; raised toilet seat; and rubber-tipped walker or cane.
3. Explain that fatigue is a common symptom of autoimmune disorders.
4. Allow the client to express feelings about altered lifestyle.
5. Help identify activities client should perform and what can be delegated. Instruct client to record level of fatigue and activities performed on an hourly basis for 24 hours. One method uses 0 to 10 scale (0 = not tired, peppy; 10 = totally exhausted).

Systemic Lupus Erythematosus

Systemic lupus erythematous (SLE) is a chronic, progressive, incurable autoimmune disease affecting multiple body organs.

Nursing Interventions

Nursing interventions for a client with SLE may include the following:

1. Warn client that sunlight and ultraviolet rays increase symptoms and tanning sessions are contraindicated.
2. Encourage client to wear protective clothing, sunscreen of at least SPF 15, and sunglasses. In cold weather, client should wear a hat and gloves.
3. Encourage client in regular oral care to promote healing of mouth sores.
4. Encourage client to visit the physician on a regular basis to monitor for early symptoms of major organ involvement.
5. Advise client to have regular eye exam if taking Plaquenil Sulfate.
6. Inform client of community support groups available through the Lupus Foundation of America, Inc.

Myasthenia Gravis

Myasthenia gravis (MG) is an autoimmune disease characterized by extreme muscle weakness and fatigue due to the body's inability to transmit nerve impulses to voluntary muscles.

Nursing Interventions

Nursing interventions for a client with MG may include the following:

1. Monitor client's respiratory rate and rhythm and breath sounds frequently.
2. Administer oxygen as ordered.

NURSING CARE OF THE CLIENT: HIV AND AIDS

CHAPTER 23

HIV TESTING

Although physicians are responsible for client counseling, the nurse must know the information to be able to answer questions and clarify the client's knowledge. Pretest counseling should include the following:

- Ask why the client believes the test should be done.
- Explain the meaning of a positive or negative test result and the possibility of a false-negative result.
- Discuss risk reduction and ways to modify behavior.
- Share state reporting requirements.
- Ensure confidentiality of test results.
- Explain that there is often stress related to test results and possible reactions to learning the results, such as depression or anxiety.
- Discuss the potential negative social consequences of positive results.
- Assist the client in making a decision about testing.
- Arrange a return appointment for the client to receive test results.

Posttest counseling should include the following:

- Review the test results with the client.
- Assess the client's understanding of the test results.
- Allow the client to express feelings about the test results.
- Review routes of HIV transmission.
- Assess the client's psychological condition including the risk for suicide.
- Assess the client's risk behavior and strategies for reducing risk.
- Provide information about support groups and national/local resources.

PULMONARY OPPORTUNISTIC INFECTIONS

Pneumocystis carinii Pneumonia

Pneumocystis carinii pneumonia (PCP) is the most common opportunistic infection associated with advanced HIV disease. Although *Pneumocystis carinii* is found primarily in the lungs, it has also been reported in the adrenal glands, bone marrow, skin, thyroid, kidneys, and spleen of persons with AIDS.

Histoplasmosis

Histoplasmosis is an infection caused by the fungus *Histoplasma capsulatum*. In most clients with HIV disease, histoplasmosis is disseminated (spread out). Histoplasmosis should be suspected if the person presents with fever of uncertain origin, cough, and malaise.

Tuberculosis

Mycobacterium tuberculosis, an acid-fast aerobic bacterium, is the cause of tuberculosis (TB). It is spread through airborne particles and enters the body by inhalation.

Nursing Interventions

Nursing interventions for the HIV-positive client with pulmonary disorders may include the following:

1. Administer 2.5–3 L of fluid per day (oral or IV) to decrease thick secretions.
2. Administer oxygen as ordered.
3. Encourage use of incentive spirometer, if not contraindicated.

GASTROINTESTINAL OPPORTUNISTIC INFECTIONS

Mycobacterium Avium Complex

Mycobacterium avium and *Mycobacterium intracellulare* are two closely related mycobacteria that are grouped together and called *Mycobacterium avium* complex (MAC). For humans, the source of exposure to MAC is contaminated water although it has been isolated from soil, dust, sediments, and aerosols.

Cytomegalovirus

Cytomegalovirus (CMV) belongs to the herpes virus group. The virus lies dormant in tissues waiting to be reactivated in the immunocompromised client. CMV causes disease by destroying the brain, lung, retina, and liver.

Cryptosporidiosis

Cryptosporidium, a protozoan causing cryptosporidiosis, usually infects the epithelial cells that line the digestive tract.

Hepatitis

Hepatitis viruses commonly seen with HIV infection are hepatitis B virus (HBV), hepatitis C virus (HCV), and hepatitis D virus (HDV).

HIV-Wasting Syndrome

HIV-wasting syndrome is defined as unexplained weight loss of more than 10% of body weight accompanied by weakness, chronic diarrhea, and fever in those infected with HIV.

Nursing Interventions

Nursing interventions for the HIV-positive client with gastrointestinal disorders may include the following:

1. Suggest client use hard candy or chewing gum to stimulate saliva production if mouth is dry.
2. Encourage client to drink liquids between (not with) meals.
3. Monitor and record intake and output.
4. Monitor client for evidence of electrolyte imbalance (hypokalemia, hypochloremia, confusion, muscle weakness).
5. Administer antiemetics and antidiarrheals as ordered.
6. Monitor stool for presence of blood, fat, undigested food.
7. Protect the perirectal area by keeping it clean and using compounds such as Aloe Vesta cream.

NURSING CARE OF THE CLIENT: MUSCULOSKELETAL SYSTEM

ASSESSMENT

Inspect and palpate to evaluate bone integrity, posture, joint function, muscle strength, and gait. Assess the client's ability to perform basic activities of daily living.

Note deformities, body alignment, abnormal growths, shortened extremities, amputations, abnormal angulation, and crepitus.

Note differences in the height of the shoulders or iliac crests. Gluteal folds should appear symmetrical. The vertebral column should be straight and perpendicular to the floor with the spine convex through the thoracic portion and concave through the cervical/lumbar portion.

Assessment of the articular system includes: range of motion (limited, active, and passive), stability of joints, deformities and any nodular formation, and pulses in the extremities.

Assess the client's ability to change position, muscle strength and coordination, and the size of individual muscles.

Examine joints for excessive fluid.

Palpate pulse points in the extremities for weak or absent pulses. Check capillary refill.

Fracture

A fracture is a break in the continuity of a bone.

Nursing Interventions

Nursing interventions for a client with musculoskeletal trauma may include the following:

1. For the client in a cast, check the edges of the cast for roughness, keep the exposed skin next to the cast clean and dry.
2. Inspect all body pressure points including the head, ears, and heels; turn the client as orders direct; and check for friction rubs.
3. Assist client in performing ROM exercises.
4. Assist client in use of adaptive devices.

Neurovascular Assessment

- Circulation, movement, and sensation (CMS) assessments are performed on clients following musculoskeletal trauma; after surgery, if nerve or blood vessel damage is possible; and following casting, splinting, and bandaging.

- The CMS assessment is performed every 15 to 30 minutes for several hours, and then every 3 to 4 hours.
- All findings must be documented.
- Tingling and numbness may be relieved by flexing fingers or toes or repositioning extremity.
- The nurse should remember 5 Ps when performing a CMS assessment:
  1. Pain
  2. Pallor (slow capillary return)
  3. Paresthesia (unrelieved tingling or numbness)
  4. Puffiness (edema)
  5. Pulselessness

Compartment Syndrome

Compartment syndrome is a form of neurovascular impairment that may lead to permanent injury of an affected limb caused by the progressive constriction of blood vessels and nerves. It can occur with any orthopedic injury as a result of bleeding into the tissue, tissue edema, or pressure from a cast or tight dressing. If untreated, in 4 to 6 hours it may lead to irreversible damage to nerves and muscles and within 24 to 48 hours permanent loss of normal limb function.

Osteomyelitis

Osteomyelitis is the inflammation of the bone and bone marrow.

Nursing Interventions

Nursing interventions for a client with osteomyelitis may include the following:

1. Handle the affected extremity gently, protect it from injury, keep it in good body alignment and level with the body.
2. Irrigate wound as ordered.
3. Use aseptic technique when irrigating the affected area and when changing the dressing.
4. Assess skin and bony prominences for reddened areas.
5. Encourage adequate fluid intake.
6. Protect client from jerky movements and falls.

Degenerative Joint Disease (Osteoarthritis)

Degenerative joint disease (DJD) is characterized by the slow and steady progressive destructive changes of the joint.

Nursing Interventions

Nursing interventions for a client with osteoarthritis may include the following:

1. Handle the affected extremity gently.
2. Coordinate with physical therapy and assist in a planned exercise program as ordered.

Total Joint Arthroplasty

Joint replacement or arthroplasty is the replacement of both articular surfaces within a joint capsule.

TOTAL HIP REPLACEMENT

Total hip replacement is the replacement of a severely damaged hip with an artificial joint.

Nursing Interventions

Following a total hip replacement the client's hip and leg should be kept in a position of abduction and extension. The knees are kept apart by using foam wedges, several pillows, or an abductor pillow. The client may lie on the unaffected side. When the client turns from the back to a side-lying position, the entire leg should be supported with pillows to keep the hip abducted. Instruct the client to avoid acute flexion of the hip. The legs should not be crossed nor the hips flexed. A raised toilet seat should be used. Vital signs and circulation, movement, and sensation (CMS) checks should be done routinely.

Dressings should be inspected frequently. If the surgical site is drained with a portable suction device, it should be monitored for patency, and the type and amount of drainage.

Inform the client to avoid hip flexion of more than 90 degrees.

TOTAL KNEE REPLACEMENT

Following total knee replacement surgery, clients may use a continuous passive motion (CPM) machine.

Following knee arthroplasty, the client's knee may be immobilized with a firm compression dressing and an adjustable soft knee immobilizer. Transfer the client out of bed to a wheelchair with the immobilizer in place. No weight bearing is allowed on the knee until it is prescribed by the surgeon.

MUSCULOSKELETAL DISORDERS

Amputations

An amputation is the removal of all or part of an extremity.

Nursing Interventions

Nursing interventions for the client who has an amputation may include the following:

1. Inspect the incision for any inflammation, excessive drainage, edema, increased pain, and hypersensitivity to touch.
2. Use aseptic technique for all dressing changes.

Carpal Tunnel Syndrome

Carpal tunnel syndrome occurs when the median nerve in the wrist is compressed by inflamed, edematous flexor tendons and tenosynovium.

Nursing Interventions

Nursing interventions for a client with carpal tunnel syndrome may include the following:

1. Encourage client to wear wrist brace.
2. Encourage client to refrain from repetitive hand movements.
3. Teach client to do ROM exercises, and to prevent twisting and turning of wrist.

NURSING CARE OF THE CLIENT: NEUROLOGICAL SYSTEM

CHAPTER 25

NEUROLOGICAL NURSING ASSESSMENT

Health History

Ask the client about headaches; clumsiness; loss of or change in function of an extremity; seizure activity; numbness or tingling; change in vision; pain; extreme fatigue; personality changes; and mood swings.

Neurological Assessment

Cerebral Function

Areas of assessment include level of consciousness, mental status, intellectual function, emotional status, pupil reaction, and communication.

The Glasgow Coma Scale is an objective tool for assessing consciousness in clients, most frequently in clients with head injuries (Table 25–1).

To assess intellectual function, ask individuals to perform certain tasks, such as the following:

- Repeating a series of numbers, such as 1, 3, 7, 1
- Telling what the individual ate for breakfast

- Adding a couple of numbers, for example, 2 + 6
- Explaining a proverb such as "the early bird gets the worm"

Observe the client's affect.

PERRLA is used for documenting pupils that are equal, round, and reactive to light and that demonstrate accommodation.

COMMUNICATION Assess both written and oral communication.

Cranial Nerve Function

Cranial nerve function essentially reflects brain stem activity.

Motor Function

Neurological screening includes assessment of muscle strength, arm and leg movement, and gait. A complete motor function assessment includes evaluating muscle size, symmetry, tone, and strength; coordination; balance; and posturing.

Sensory Function

A subjective examination of sensory function, performed with the client's eyes closed, is generally done

135

only when a dysfunction is suspected. The examiner must test tactile sensation, pain and temperature, vibration, proprioception, stereognosis, graphesthesia, and integration of sensations.

Assessment of Reflexes

Refer to Table 25-2 for a reflex grading scale. The Babinski phenomenon is the most important abnormal superficial reflex. The bottom of the foot is stroked with a key, or other object, starting at the heel and moving along the lateral side of the sole, then moving toward the big toe. The normal adult response is a slight plantar flexion or curling under of the toes. An abnormal response is dorsal flexion and fanning of the toes. This phenomena indicates corticospinal disease in people with mature central nervous systems.

Table 25-1 GLASGOW COMA SCALE

BEHAVIOR	RESPONSE	SCORE
Eye opening response	Spontaneous	4
	To verbal command	3
	To pain	2
	No response	1
Best verbal response	Oriented, conversing	5
	Disoriented, conversing	4
	Use of inappropriate words	3
	Incomprehensible sounds	2
	No response	1
Best motor response	Obeys verbal commands	6
	Moves to localized pain	5
	Flexion withdrawal to pain	4
	Abnormal posturing—decorticate	3
	Abnormal posturing—decerebrate	2
	No response	1
Total		3 to 15

Table 25-2 REFLEX GRADING SCALE

GRADE	DEFINITION
4	Hyperactive with clonus (alternating muscle contractions between antagonistic muscles)
3	Hyperactive
2	Normal
1	Hypoactive
0	Absent

HEAD INJURY

Head injuries involve trauma to the scalp, skull, or brain.

BRAIN INJURY

Brain injuries are caused by primary injuries of acceleration–deceleration force, rotational force, or penetrating missile.

Nursing Interventions

Nursing interventions for a client with a head injury may include the following:

1. Assess neurological status of client every 15 to 60 minutes. Note findings on Glasgow Coma Scale. Compare findings to previous assessments to uncover changes in condition.
2. Position client with head of the bed up 30° to 40° and client's head at midline to promote venous drainage from the head.
3. Assess respiratory status every 15 to 60 minutes.
4. Continually assess ABG levels or pulse oximeter readings.
5. Administer oxygen as ordered.
6. Teach small segments of information at a time and reinforce teaching.
7. Assess communication deficits.
8. Allow time for the client to attempt to communicate needs.
9. Anticipate needs to prevent client frustration in trying to communicate.
10. Use gestures, pictures, and closed questions (those requiring only a "yes" or "no" answer).
11. Provide paper and pencil if dominant side is unaffected.
12. Adapt environment to prevent injury of the client with unilateral neglect by positioning water and personal items on the unaffected or unneglected side.
13. Approach the client from the un-neglected side.
14. Place small bites of food on unaffected side and check for food in the cheek on the affected side after meals.

Epilepsy/Seizure Disorder

Epilepsy is a disorder of cerebral function in which the client experiences sudden attacks of altered consciousness, motor activity, or sensory phenomenon. Convulsive seizures are the most common type of attack.

Nursing Interventions

Nursing interventions for a client with a seizure may include the following:

1. Following tonic–clonic activity, turn client to the side to allow secretions to drain from the airway.
2. Assess skin color and respiratory rate and depth during and following seizure.
3. Administer oxygen as needed.
4. During seizures in bed, use blankets or protective pads to pad side rails.
5. If client is standing or sitting, ease client to the floor when seizure activity begins.
6. Teach client about ways of maintaining a safe environment, including driving restrictions; lying down in a safe area if an aura is experienced; showering instead

of tub bathing; either avoiding swimming or swimming with a partner if the physician allows; and wearing a medical identification tag.

Herniated Intervertebral Disk

In herniation, or rupture of the disk, the nucleus pulposus protrudes, pressing on the spinal cord and nerve roots, causing pain, motor changes, sensory changes, and alterations in reflexes.

Nursing Interventions

Nursing interventions for a client with a herniated intervertebral disk may include the following:

1. Assess pain intensity and location, as well as activities or position when pain began. Have the client rate pain on a scale of 1 to 10.
2. Place client in position of comfort, usually on back, with knees slightly flexed and a small pillow beneath head, or on unaffected side, with affected extremity flexed and a pillow between the legs.
3. Apply moist heat as prescribed and administer medications to relieve pain, relax muscles, and relieve inflammation and anxiety, as ordered. Document effectiveness.

Spinal Cord Injury

Spinal cord injury (SCI) occurs from trauma to the spinal cord or from compression of the spinal cord due to injury to the supporting structures.

Nursing Interventions

Nursing interventions for the client with a spinal cord injury in the subacute phase of care may include the following:

1. Assess the client's risk factors for additional injury.
2. Use enough personnel to turn client correctly to maintain alignment of client's spinal column.
3. Provide routine care for halo device by opening vest on one side to cleanse skin under vest at least daily and to assess for skin breakdown. Repeat procedure on the other side.
4. Monitor pin sites of halo device every shift for placement.
5. Perform pin site care using facility protocol.
6. Teach client causes and symptoms of autonomic dysreflexia: increased blood pressure, sudden throbbing headache, chills, pallor, goose flesh, nausea, and/or metallic taste in mouth.
7. Observe for bradycardia, vasodilatation, flushing, and diaphoresis above the level of spinal cord injury. If these symptoms occur, immediately notify the physician and administer medications as ordered to decrease blood pressure. Raise head of bed and lower legs to reduce blood pressure. Then, remove the noxious stimuli, which may include constrictive clothing, shoes, splints, or linens.

Parkinson's Disease

Parkinson's disease is a chronic, progressive, degenerative disease affecting the area of the brain controlling movement.

Nursing Interventions

Nursing interventions for a client with Parkinson's disease may include the following:

1. Assess degree of muscle involvement by testing ROM, muscular rigidity, tremors, and gait.
2. Administer medications within the time window that provides a constant therapeutic level for symptom control.
3. Perform passive and active ROM exercises to maintain function.
4. Ambulate, as client is able to tolerate.
5. Frequently turn client in bed.
6. Assess client's ability to perform selfcare.
7. Encourage client to perform as much self-care as possible.
8. Consult with occupational therapy for methods to increase the ability to perform self-care.
9. Assist with daily care that the client is unable to perform alone.
10. Position client sitting upright when eating.
11. Position client's head slightly forward and never extended to facilitate swallowing.

Multiple Sclerosis

Multiple sclerosis (MS) is a chronic, progressive, degenerative disease wherein scattered nerve cells of the brain and spinal cord are demyelinated.

Nursing Interventions

Nursing interventions for a client with MS may include the following:

1. Assess motor status every 4 to 24 hours.
2. Provide active and passive ROM every 8 hours.

3. Turn bedridden clients every 2 hours.
4. Use pillows, splints, high-topped (above the ankles) shoes with laces to maintain proper body alignment.
   Encourage client to perform daily activities as able given the limitations of the disease.
5. Ambulate client four times daily with use of assistive devices as necessary.
6. Assess for bladder retention, incontinence, or urinary tract infection.
7. Maintain fluid intake of 1,000 cc/day.
8. Assess client's concept of self in relation to changes brought about by the disease process.

Amyotrophic Lateral Sclerosis (Lou Gehrig's Disease)

Amyotrophic lateral sclerosis (ALS) is a progressive, fatal disease characterized by the degeneration of motor neurons in the cortex, medulla, and spinal cord.

Nursing Interventions

Nursing interventions for a client with ALS may include the following:

1. Assess breath sounds for presence of congestion; skin for pressure areas; and legs for thrombophlebitis.
2. Prolong verbal communication with speech therapy interventions consisting of voice projection and speech devices.
3. Develop alternate methods of communicating prior to the loss of verbal skills.

4. Assess breathing patterns frequently and observe for aspiration and the loss of the swallow reflex.
5. Turn from side to side to allow oral secretions to drain from mouth; suction oral pharynx, as necessary.

Alzheimer's Disease

Alzheimer's disease (AD) is a progressive, degenerative neurological disease wherein brain cells are destroyed. The cerebral cortex atrophies, and neuron loss and changes within the brain cells occur.

Nursing Interventions

Nursing interventions for the client with Alzheimer's may include the following:

1. Assess client's ability to perceive environmental hazards.
2. Maintain a safe environment: eliminate clutter, position furniture/equipment in same place, monitor temperature of hot water and food, maintain monitoring system to prevent wandering into adverse climate or into traffic, provide adequate lighting, orient client and family to surroundings and reorient as necessary.
3. Develop memory aids and cues to help client remember.
4. Maintain a consistent environment and daily schedule.
5. Approach client in a quiet, nonthreatening manner.
6. Attend to nonverbal cues for unmet needs (e.g., pacing, grimacing, crying, agitation). The client may be

hungry, have a full bladder, or be unable to ask to be repositioned.
7. Give simple, single instructions.
8. Advise the client to avoid caffeine.

GUILLAIN-BARRÉ SYNDROME (POLYRADICULO-NEUROPATHY)

Guillain-Barré syndrome is an acute inflammatory process primarily involving the motor neurons of the peripheral nervous system.

Nursing Interventions

Nursing interventions for a client with Guillain-Barré syndrome may include the following:

1. Administer oxygen as ordered.
2. Provide mechanical ventilation for respiratory failure.
3. Perform respiratory assessment for diminished breath sounds or congestion.
4. Assess for calf tenderness, redness, or increased warmth.
5. Use plexipulse boots.
6. Initiate rehabilitation following acute phase of illness with strengthening exercises, occupational therapy, and getting client out of bed several times per day to build strength and endurance.

Encephalitis, Meningitis

Encephalitis is inflammation of the brain. Meningitis is inflammation of the meninges. The most common cause of encephalitis or meningitis is a virus.

Nursing Interventions

1. Monitor for changes in neurological status, especially for changes in level of consciousness and for signs of increasing intracranial pressure.
2. Observed for seizure activity and protect from injury.
3. Administer analgesics for relief of headaches.

Huntington's Disease or Chorea

Huntington's disease is a chronic, progressive hereditary disease of the nervous system. It is characterized by a progressive involuntary choreiform movement and progressive dementia.

Nursing Interventions

1. Teach the client and family about the disease process, the progress of the disease, and the genetic factors involved.

Gilles de la Tourette's Syndrome

Gilles de la Tourette's syndrome is a neurological movement disorder that also has prominent behavioral manifestations.

Nursing Interventions

1. Inform the client and the family about the availability of support groups for clients with Tourette's syndrome.
2. Teach about the disease process and expectations for the client.

NURSING CARE OF THE CLIENT: SENSORY SYSTEM

CHAPTER 26

ASSESSMENT

The physical examination focuses specifically on the client's ability to hear, see, taste, smell, and touch (Table 26–1).

Cataracts

A cataract is a disorder that causes the lens or its capsule to lose its transparency and/or become opaque.

Nursing Interventions

Nursing interventions for a client with cataracts may include the following:

1. Teach the client to avoid reaching for objects to maintain stability when ambulating, as depth perception is altered.
2. Discuss the client's ability to meet self-care needs and activities of daily living.

Retinal Detachment

Retinal detachment is an actual separation of the retina from the choroid.

Nursing Interventions

Nursing interventions for a client with retinal detachment may include the following:

1. Assess degree and duration of visual impairment.
2. Explain surgery routines. Postoperative: Positioning (supine with a small pillow under the head), bilateral eye patches, activity restrictions, and need to call for assistance with ambulation until stable and vision is adequate.

Injury

Injuries to the eyes require immediate attention by an ophthalmologist. Even a few hours delay in treatment may lead to permanent damage.

Corneal abrasion is the disruption of cells and the loss of the superficial epithelium.

FOREIGN BODIES

Foreign bodies often become embedded in the conjunctiva under the

Table 26-1 ASSESSING SENSORY PERCEPTUAL STATUS

SENSATION BEING ASSESSED	ASSESSMENT FOCUS
Visual	• Presence of visual problems, including: —Decreased acuity —Blurred vision —Double vision —Blind spots —Rainbows or halos around objects —Photosensitivity —Loss of peripheral field (narrowing) • Difficulty seeing far or near • Family history of visual problems (such as glaucoma, cataracts) • Use of contact lenses or eyeglasses • Date of last eye examination
Auditory	• Presence of hearing problems • Recent changes in hearing ability • Ability to distinguish sounds (tone and pitch) • Presence of buzzing or ringing noises • Use of a hearing aid
Gustatory	• Changes in ability to taste • Difficulty in differentiating salty, sweet, sour, and bitter tastes • Changes in appetite
Olfactory	• Changes in ability to smell • Ability to distinguish common smells (such as food, perfume, flowers)
Tactile	• Difficulty in feeling temperature changes in extremities • Impairment of pain perception in extremities • Presence of unusual sensations in extremities (such as tingling or numbness)

upper eyelid. The lid must be everted and the client instructed to look up to facilitate inspection and removal. If the particle is not located and removed, sterile fluorescein drops or strips should be instilled to visualize minute foreign bodies not readily visible with the naked eye.

CHEMICAL BURNS

Emergency treatment of chemical burns to the conjunctiva or cornea includes immediate lavage of the eye with tap water and referral to an emergency room or ophthalmologist. In the emergency room, a specially made lid speculum is placed directly on the eyeball and connected to a minimum of one liter of isotonic saline solution for irrigation. A topical anesthetic may be instilled to minimize pain during irrigation. No attempt should be made to neutralize the chemical, since the heat generated by the chemical reaction may cause further injury. Both eyes should then be patched to allow more comfort.

NURSING CARE OF THE CLIENT: ENDOCRINE SYSTEM

CHAPTER 27

Diabetes Mellitus

Diabetes mellitus is a disorder of metabolism. Insulin is a hormone produced and secreted by the beta cells in the islets of Langerhans of the pancreas. Insulin stimulates the active transport of glucose into muscle and adipose tissue cells, making it available for cell use. For glucose to cross the cell membrane, insulin must connect with a receptor on the cell membrane. Some clients with diabetes mellitus have enough insulin, but too few functioning receptor sites. Others have inadequate or no insulin production.

The amount of glucose in the blood regulates the rate of insulin secretion. When a meal is eaten, the blood glucose elevates and the beta cells of the islets of Langerhans release insulin. As the blood glucose level drops, insulin secretion diminishes.

Insulin actively promotes those processes that lower the blood glucose level and inhibits those processes that raise the blood glucose level. A deficiency of insulin results in hyperglycemia, or elevated blood glucose. Excess insulin results in hypoglycemia (low blood glucose). Diabetes mellitus is a group of disorders characterized by chronic hyperglycemia.

DIAGNOSIS AND CLASSIFICATION

The following criteria were developed by the Expert Committee on the Diagnosis and Classification of Diabetes Mellitus (1997).

Diagnosis

Two precursors to diabetes have been identified.

1. Impaired glucose tolerance (IGT) —a glucose level of 140 to 199 mg/dL 2 hours after a glucose load

2. Impaired fasting glucose (IFG)— a fasting glucose of 110 to 125 mg/dL

Classification

Type 1 Diabetes

There are two forms of diabetes resulting from pancreatic beta-cell destruction or a primary defect in beta-cell function resulting in no release of insulin and ineffective glucose transport. There is usually an absolute insulin deficiency so the clients are insulin-dependent. The two subdivisions of type 1 diabetes are:

- Immune-mediated—islet cell or insulin antibodies destroy beta cells.
- Idiopathic—no evidence of autoimmunity; the individual just does not produce insulin and is prone to ketoacidosis.

Type 2 Diabetes

These clients have insulin resistance with relative insulin deficiency. Most of these clients are obese.

Insulin

Persons with type 1 diabetes always require insulin administration. Persons with type 2 diabetes often do not require insulin when initially diagnosed, but insulin therapy may become necessary over time, as endogenous insulin production decreases, or during times of stress or illness (Table 27–1).

Acute Complications of Diabetes

There are three major acute complications of diabetes related to blood glucose imbalance: hypoglycemia, diabetic ketoacidosis (DKA), and hyperglycemic hyperosmolar nonketotic syndrome (HHNK) (Table 27–2).

Hypoglycemia (Insulin Reaction)

Hypoglycemia (low blood glucose) occurs when a client's glucose level drops below 70 mg/dL, with the most severe reactions occurring when it drops below 50 mg/dL.

Diabetic Ketoacidosis

Diabetic ketoacidosis (DKA) is one of the most serious complications of hyperglycemia.

Hyperglycemic Hyperosmolar Nonketotic Syndrome

Hyperglycemic hyperosmolar nonketotic (HHNK) syndrome occurs when there is insufficient insulin to

Table 27–1 TYPES OF INSULIN AND THEIR ACTIONS

TYPES OF INSULIN	APPEARANCE	ACTION IN HOURS		
		ONSET	PEAK	DURATION
Very short-acting insulin Lispro (Humalog)	clear	1/4	1–1 1/2	5 or less
Short-acting Humulin R	clear	1/2–1	2–4	6–8
Intermediate-acting Humulin U	cloudy	1–1 1/2	4–12	up to 24
Humulin L	cloudy	1–2–1/2	7–15	22
Long-acting Humulin U	cloudy	4–8	10–30	36+
Premixed Reg/Humulin N Humulin 70/30 Humulin 50/50	cloudy	1/2–1	4–8	24

Table 27–2 SYMPTOMS OF ACUTE COMPLICATIONS OF DIABETES

SYMPTOMS OF HYPOGLYCEMIA (INSULIN REACTION)

Mild hypoglycemia

- Diaphoresis
- Pallor
- Paresthesias
- Excess hunger
- Palpitations
- Tremors
- Anxiety

Moderate hypoglycemia

- Confusion, disorientation
- Slurred speech
- Behavior changes
- Irritability

Severe hypoglycemia

- Seizures
- Loss of consciousness
- Shallow respirations
- Nursing Alert: Severe hypoglycemia is a medical emergency. Administer some form of glucose immediately.

SYMPTOMS OF DIABETIC KETOACIDOSIS (DKA)

- Same as HHNK plus symptoms of acidosis:
- "Fruity" odor to breath
- Kussmaul's respirations (deep, nonlabored)
- Nausea and vomiting
- Headache

SYMPTOMS OF HYPERGLYCEMIC HYPEROSMOLAR NONKETOTIC (HHNK) SYNDROME

- Polyuria
- Polydipsia
- Skin hot, dry, decreased turgor
- Dehydration—hypotension, increased pulse
- Blurred vision
- Weakness
- Mental status changes, confusion to coma

---

prevent hyperglycemia, but enough insulin to prevent ketoacidosis.

Blood glucose level ranges from 600 to 2,000 mg/dL and serum osmolality > 350 mOsm/L.

Nursing Interventions

Nursing interventions for a client with diabetes mellitus may include the following:

1. Teach client about diabetes and the use of insulin to prevent hyper-/hypoglycemia or assist client to enroll in a formal diabetic education program.
2. Teach client about oral hypoglycemics or insulin, whichever the client will be using.
3. Discuss how exercise is related to diabetes management.
4. Discuss how dietary management is related to the control of blood glucose and provide an exchange list of foods.
5. Teach client how to perform SMBG and have client return demonstration.
6. Provide client with a list of symptoms and treatment for hypoglycemia.

Syndrome of Inappropriate Antidiuretic Hormone

Syndrome of inappropriate antidiuretic hormone (SIADH) results from an excess of ADH. This causes the kidneys to reabsorb excess water, which decreases urine output and increases fluid volume.

Nursing Interventions

Nursing interventions for a client with SIADH may include the following:

1. Assess client's weight daily on same scale at same time.
2. Accurately record I & O.
3. Maintain fluid restrictions.
4. Provide frequent oral care.
5. Allow client to rinse mouth with water, but not swallow any.

6. Provide lubricant for client's lips.
7. Allow client to choose fluids and times to drink them.

Diabetes Insipidus

Diabetes insipidus is a deficiency of ADH, causing a metabolic disorder characterized by severe polyuria and polydipsia.

Nursing Interventions

Nursing interventions for a client with diabetes insipidus may include the following:

1. Monitor the client for dizziness and weakness. Record client intake and output.
2. Provide fluids as ordered to cover output.
3. Monitor weight daily.
4. Provide oral care. Use a soft toothbrush, mild mouthwash, and lubricant for the lips.
5. Assess condition of oral mucous membranes.
6. Encourage adequate intake of fluids, protein, vitamin C, and calories.

Cancer of the Thyroid

Cancer of the thyroid is rare and occurs in all age groups. Individuals who have had radiation therapy to the neck are more susceptible.

Nursing Interventions

Nursing interventions for the client with thyroid cancer may involve the following:

1. Monitor the client's level of anxiety.
2. Encourage the client to discuss feelings about the diagnosis and possible surgery.
3. Assist the client in identifying previously successful coping methods.
4. Teach new coping methods if needed.

Addison's Disease (Adrenal Hypofunction)

Addison's disease, primary hypofunctioning of the adrenals, involves decreased functioning of the adrenal cortex and its secretions—mineralocorticoids, glucocorticoids, and androgens.

Nursing Interventions

Nursing interventions for the client with Addison's disease may include the following:

1. Monitor the client's vital signs, level of consciousness, intake and output, and weight.
2. Administer IV fluids as ordered and encourage fluid intake.
3. Monitor temperature every 4 hours unless elevated, then every 2 hours.
4. Provide a private room with reverse or protective isolation as needed.

NURSING CARE OF THE CLIENT: GASTROINTESTINAL SYSTEM

ASSESSMENT

For clients complaining of GI symptoms, the assessment should include:

1. History of the present complaint including length and frequency of symptoms, when symptoms occur, as well as aggravating factors.

2. Medication history including prescribed and over-the-counter (OTC) medications, and their effectiveness.

3. A complete nutritional history; a note should be made of any foods that increase or decrease symptoms. Also, assess if meals aggravate symptoms or if symptoms occur within a specific time period after a meal. Note the fiber and fat content of the diet as well as the amount of fluids typically consumed.

4. Psychosocial factors including meal patterns should be evaluated: note if the client eats alone, eats large meals at regular intervals, or snacks all day.

5. Physical examination including inspection, auscultation, percussion, and palpation of the abdomen. An evaluation of the client's ability to chew and swallow is also important.

6. Bowel elimination patterns including frequency, consistency, and amounts of bowel movements.

7. Evaluation of diagnostic data.

Esophageal Varices

A varix is an enlarged, tortuous vein or, occasionally, an artery. The varices are often associated with cirrhosis of the liver or any other condition that causes chronic obstruction of drainage from the esophageal veins into the portal veins.

Nursing Interventions

Nursing interventions for a client with esophageal varices may include the following:

1. Monitor vital signs every 4 hours including orthostatic blood pressures.

2. Monitor for nausea and dizziness.

3. Monitor H & H.

Gastroesophageal Reflux Disease

Gastroesophageal reflux disease (GERD) is a disease in which the gastric secretions flow upward into the esophagus, damaging the tissues. An inability of the lower esophageal sphincter (LES) to close fully contributes to this condition.

Nursing Interventions

1. Encourage weight loss as needed.
2. Teach the client to avoid fatty foods, alcohol, nicotine, caffeine, and spicy foods.
3. Administer medications as instructed.
4. Teach the client to sleep with the head of the bed elevated 2 to 4 inches on blocks.
5. Advise the client to avoid wearing constrictive clothing.

Ulcers

Peptic ulcers are erosions that form in the esophagus, stomach, or duodenum resulting from acid/pepsin imbalance. Gastric ulcers refer to erosions in the stomach.

Nursing Interventions

Nursing interventions for a client with ulcers may include the following:

1. Check vital signs every 4 hours and PRN including orthostatic blood pressure.
2. Administer IV fluids, electrolyte replacement, and blood transfusions as ordered.
3. Monitor for dizziness and nausea.
4. Check stool for blood.

Appendicitis

Appendicitis is the inflammation of the vermiform appendix, a 10-cm small, slender tube attached to the cecum.

Nursing Interventions

Nursing interventions for the client with appendicitis may include the following:

1. Preoperatively, monitor client's pain.
2. Check abdomen for rigidity.
3. Provide an ice pack to help relieve pain as ordered; never use heat.
4. Postoperatively, give analgesics as ordered and medicate prior to activities such as ambulation.
   Teach client to use a pillow to splint the incision when coughing.
5. If client is having difficulty passing flatus, administer enemas or a rectal tube as ordered, and encourage ambulation.
6. If adhesive strips are present, leave in place until they no longer cover the incision (approximately 10 days to 2 weeks).

Inflammatory Bowel Disease

Inflammatory bowel disease (IBD) is the term used to describe Crohn's disease and ulcerative colitis (UC). Crohn's disease is characterized by lesions that affect the entire thickness of the bowel and can occur anywhere throughout the colon and small intestine.

UC is characterized by mucosal lesions occurring typically in the rectal area and sigmoid colon and progressing throughout the colon.

Surgical Management

In severe cases of UC resistant to medical management, the colon is removed and an ileostomy is performed, curing the disease. (Refer to Stomal/Ostomy management in section following) Most clients with Crohn's disease need surgery at some point to repair the structural damage caused by scarring. Intestinal obstructions and perforations may also occur in Crohn's disease, necessitating further surgery. Surgical intervention, however, does not cure the disease.

Nursing Interventions

Nursing interventions for clients with Crohn's disease or UC may include the following:

1. Monitor I & O every shift; caloric count and weight daily.
2. Administer IV fluid and electrolyte replacement as ordered.
3. Provide high-calorie, high-protein supplements as ordered along with small, frequent meals.
4. Administer TPN. Closely monitor lab reports for electrolytes and glucose level.

Stomal/Ostomy Management

On return from surgery, the new stoma will be edematous and range from deep red to dusky in color.

Nursing Interventions

Nursing interventions for clients with ostomies may include:

1. Check the color of the stoma with a penlight and document at least once a shift.
2. Call the physician if the stoma becomes black.
3. Monitor bowel function every shift for any obstruction or ileus.
4. Check bowel sounds, distention, and abdominal tenderness every 4 hours.
5. Check the incision and stoma site for bleeding.
6. Check the blood pressure and pulse frequently after surgery.

Peritonitis

Peritonitis is the inflammation of the peritoneum, the membranous covering of the abdomen.

Nursing Interventions

Nursing interventions for a client with peritonitis may include the following:

1. Monitor I & O every shift.
2. Monitor for dehydration: decrease in urine output, dry mucous membranes, and poor skin turgor.
3. Monitor NG tube to decompress abdomen. Maintain patency of NG tube.

Cirrhosis

Cirrhosis refers to the chronic, degenerative changes in the liver cells and thickening of surrounding tissue that result from the liver repairing itself after chronic inflammation.

If portal hypertension cannot be controlled with medications, a portosystemic shunt or a transjugular intrahepatic portosystemic shunt (TIPS) may be performed. The purpose of the shunt is to redirect the blood flow, thereby relieving the portal hypertension and decreasing the risk of rupturing distended veins in the esophagus.

Nursing Interventions

Nursing interventions for a client with cirrhosis may include the following:

1. Weigh daily.
2. Measure abdominal girth daily.
3. Restrict fluid to 1,000 to 2,000 cc per day.
4. Administer tap water enemas and lactulose as ordered to eliminate ammonia-rich stools.
5. Monitor ammonia levels.
6. Provide low protein diet.

Hepatitis

Hepatitis is a chronic or acute inflammation of the liver caused by a virus, bacteria, drugs, alcohol abuse, or other toxic substances. Refer to Table 28-1 for a comparison of different types of viral hepatitis.

Nursing Interventions

Nursing interventions for the client with hepatitis may include the following:

1. For clients with hepatitis A, teach client to disinfect articles contaminated with feces (such as the toilet), not to prepare food for others, and not to share articles such as eating utensils or toothbrushes.
2. For clients with hepatitis B, teach to avoid sexual contact until they test negative for HBsAg or their partners are immunized with the HBV vaccine.
3. For clients with hepatitis C, teach that it is unknown whether it can be transmitted through sexual contact, so precautions are recommended until more is known.
4. Educate client regarding reasons for fatigue and that fatigue may be present for several months.

Pancreatitis

Pancreatitis is an acute or chronic inflammation of the pancreas caused when pancreatic enzymes digest the lining of the pancreas.

Nursing Interventions

Nursing interventions for a client with pancreatitis may include the following:

1. Monitor NG tube to decompress the abdomen.
2. Administer analgesics as ordered and monitor for relief.
3. Assess pain for increasing severity that would indicate worsening pancreatitis.
4. Monitor serum amylase, WBCs, and H & H for signs of increasing severity of pancreatitis or hemorrhage.
5. Monitor I & O every shift.

Colorectal Cancer

Almost all colorectal cancers arise from polyps, an abnormal growth of tissue that protrudes into the colon. Refer to Table 28-2 for classification and treatment of colorectal cancer.

Table 28–1 COMPARISON OF DIFFERENT TYPES OF VIRAL HEPATITIS

	A	B
Etiologic Agent	hepatitis A viris (HAV)	hepatitis B virus (HBV)
Transmission	Fecal-oral; contaminated water or food; person to person	Blood; sexual; perinatal; breast milk
Risk Groups	Household/sexual contact with infected person; international travelers	Injection drug users; Sexual/household contact with infected person; infants born to infected mothers; health care workers multiple sex partners
Incubation Period	15–50 days	45–160 days
Infectious Period	Usually less than 2 months	Before symptoms appear; lifetime if carrier
Diagnostic Tests	IgM anti-HAV	HBsAg
Symptoms	Flu-like; jaundice; dark yellow urine; light colored stools	Flu-like; may have jaundice; dark yellow urine; light colored stools
Prevention	Standard Precautions; enteric precautions; Hepatitis A vaccine (entire series); Immune globulin (for short term)	Standard Precautions; reduce risk behaviors; Hepatitis B vaccine (entire series); Immune globulin (for short term)
Treatment	Immune globulin within 2 weeks of exposure	Immune globulin (HBIg) Alpha interferon
Prognosis	Rarely fatal; not a carrier	No cure; may become a carrier

Data from: Centers for Disease Control and Prevention (CDC) (2000). Viral hepatitis A. [Online] Available: www.cdc.gov/ncidod/diseases/hepatitis/a/index.htm; CDC (2000). Viral hepatitis B. [On-line] Available: www.cdc.gov/ncidod/diseases/hepatitis/b/index.htm; CDC (2000). Viral hepatitis C. [On-line] Available: www.cdc.gov/ncidod/diseases/hepatitis/c/index.htm; CDC (2000). Viral hepatitis D. [on-line] Available: www.cdc.gov/ncidod/diseases/hepatitis/d/hep00051; CDC (2000). Viral hepatitis E. [On-line] Available: www.cdc.gov/ncidod/diseases/hepatitis/e/hep00058; Lau, D. T., Kleiner, D. E., Park, Y., DiBisceglie, A. M. & Hoofnagle, J. H. (1999). Resolution of chronic delta hepatitis after 12 years of interferon alpha therapy. Gastroenterology, 117(5), 1229–33; National Institute of

C	D	E
hepatitis C virus (HCV)	hepatitis D virus (HDV)	hepatitis E virus (HEV)
Blood	Only persons with hepatitis B can get hepatitis D; blood and blood products; needle sticks; seldom sexual; rarely perinatal	Oral-fecal route; contaminated water; person to person uncommon
Blood transfusions or organ transplants prior to 1992; sharing needles; exposure to blood and blood products	Needle sharing; needle sticks	Mainly travel to countries where endemic
14–180 days	15–60 days	15–60 days
Before symptoms appear; lifetime if carrier	Not determined	Not determined
Anti HCV; serum ALT increased 10x; HCVRNA	IgG anti-HDV	None available
Many have no symptoms; flu-like	Flu-like; may have jaundice; dark yellow urine; light colored stools	Abdominal pain, anorexia; dark yellow urine; jaundice, fever
Standard Precautions; reduce risk behaviors; no vaccine	Standard Precautions; reduce risk behaviors; Hepatitis B vaccine; if client already has hepatitis B no prevention for hepatitis D	Standard Precautions; be sure water safe when traveling; no vaccine
Alpha interferon; ribavirin (Virazole)	Alpha interferon	None given
85% or less have chronic infection; 70% develop chronic liver disease	Chronicity uncommon	No evidence of chronicity

Diabetes and Digestive and Kidney Diseases (NIDDK) (1997). What I need to know about hepatitis A [On-line] Available: www.niddk.nih.gov/health/digest/pubs/hep/hepa/hepa.htm; NIDDK (1998). What I Need to Know About Hepatitis B. [On-line] Available: www.niddk. nih.gov/health/digest/pubs/hep/hepb/hepb.htm; NIDDK (1999). What I Need to Know About Hepatitis C. [On-line] Available: www.niddk.nih.gov/health/digest/pubs/hep/hepc/hepc.htm; NIDDK (2000). Chronic hepatitis C: Current disease management. [On-line] Available: www.niddk.nih.gov/health/digest/pubs/chrnhepc/chrnhepc.htm; NIDDK (2000). The digestive diseases dictionary: E–K. [On-line] Available: www.niddk.nih.gov/health/ digest/pubs/dddctnry/pages/e-k.htm.

Table 28–2 COLORECTAL CANCER CLASSIFICATION AND TREATMENT

CLASS	INVOLVEMENT	TREATMENT
Class A	Limited to the inner lining of the colon.	Polypectomy during colonoscopy removes cancer.
Class B	Involves from 2 layers to entire thickness of colon wall.	Colon resection, chemotherapy.
Class C	Class B with invasion to lymph nodes.	Colon resection, chemotherapy, and immunotherapy.
Class D	Metastases to other organs (lung and liver most common).	Colon resection as a palliative measure only. Chemotherapy, radiation, and immunotherapy.

Nursing Interventions

Nursing interventions for a client with colorectal cancer may include the following:

1. Monitor the NG tube until bowel sounds return.
2. Ambulate the client the day of surgery or the next day.

Liver Cancer

Primary liver cancer is rare. Most liver tumors are metastatic from other sites in the body. A primary liver tumor can be removed surgically if the disease is not extensive. Metastases cannot be surgically removed and are usually treated with chemotherapy and radiation.

NURSING CARE OF THE CLIENT: URINARY SYSTEM

CHAPTER 29

ASSESSMENT

The nurse asks the client open-ended questions.

Subjective Data

Is there pain? Is it sharp or a dull ache? Constant or intermittent? Does it radiate to the groin, genital area, or leg? Is the pain associated with urination? Have headaches been experienced?

Is there difficulty starting the stream? Is there urgency, frequency, incontinence, or hematuria? Does the bladder feel empty after voiding? Does the client have pruritis or dry skin?

Objective Data

Ask the client if edema is always present or whether it disappears during the night. Monitor I & O and vital signs. Palpate the bladder for retention. Weigh the client. Assess mucous membranes for moisture and the skin for dryness and uremic frost. Evaluate urine for color, clarity, and odor.

Pyelonephritis

Pyelonephritis is a bacterial infection of the renal pelvis, tubules, and interstitial tissue of one or both kidneys.

Nursing Interventions

Nursing interventions for a client with pyelonephritis may include the following:

1. Encourage drinking of cranberry juice.
2. Encourage 3,000 mL fluid intake per day, especially water.
3. Monitor intake and output.
4. Instruct the client to take all the antimicrobial medication as prescribed in order to eliminate the bacteria.
5. Teach client to weigh daily and report sudden weight gain (2 pounds/week) to the physician.

Acute Glomerulonephritis

In both acute and chronic disease, the glomerulus within the nephron unit becomes inflamed.

Nursing Interventions

Nursing interventions for a client with acute glomerulonephritis may include the following:

1. Fluids will be restricted with specific amounts designated throughout the day. For example, 900 mL of fluids for a day might be divided in the following manner: 7 A.M. to 3 P.M. 600 mL; 3 P.M. to 11 P.M. 200 mL; 11 P.M. to 7 A.M. 100 mL.
2. Maintain accurate intake and output records hourly.
3. Advise that thirst may be relieved by sucking on hard candy or, if allowed, a few ice chips.
4. Provide eye care with normal saline to promote comfort from the periorbital edema.
5. If hematuria and/or proteinuria are still present, provide a diet with mild to moderate protein restriction to rest the kidney tissue.
6. If edema persists, provide low-sodium diet.
7. Before discharge, teach client and family about diet, fluids, and activity restrictions and measuring fluid intake and urine output.
8. Explain the importance of protecting the client from other infections.
9. Allow no one with an upper respiratory infection to visit the client.

Chronic Glomerulonephritis

Chronic glomerulonephritis is a progressive but slow, destructive process affecting the glomeruli, causing loss of kidney function.

Nursing Interventions

Nursing interventions for a client with chronic glomerulonephritis may include the following:

1. Measure urine output.
2. Assess and document the color and consistency of the urine.
3. Weigh client daily at the same time each day, on the same scale and with the same clothes.
4. Assess and describe the location of the edema.
5. Assess skin every time the client is repositioned.
6. Cleanse the skin frequently, especially when crystals of urea form on the skin, causing itching and dryness.

Urolithiasis

Urolithiasis is a calculus, or stone, formed in the urinary tract.

Nursing Interventions

Nursing interventions for a client with urolithiasis may include the following:

1. Develop a pain management plan.
2. Inquire about intensity, location, duration, and alleviating factors of pain.
3. Administer analgesics and antispasmodics as ordered.
4. Monitor urine for color and amount.
5. Encourage fluids to dilute the urine and flush out the calculi.
6. Assist client to ambulate, if able.
7. Accurately monitor intake and output.

Urinary Bladder Tumors

Benign papillomas are the most common urinary bladder tumor and should be treated aggressively because they are considered to be premalignant. Cancer cells develop mainly in the area where the ureters enter the urinary bladder.

Nursing Interventions

Nursing interventions for a client with urinary bladder tumors may include the following:

1. If surgical removal of bladder lesions is done as an outpatient procedure, teach the client to observe for pink-tinged urine and to notify the physician if bright red urine is seen.
2. Accurately monitor urine output.

Renal Tumors

A unilateral renal adenocarcinoma is the most common tumor and is seen more often in men between the ages of 50 and 70.

Nursing Interventions

Nursing interventions for a client with renal tumors may include the following:

1. Inform the client of the assessments to be done: neurological status, lung sounds, the incision, Homans' sign, peripheral pulses, vital signs, and serum electrolyte values.
2. Teach the importance of accurate intake and output records.

Polycystic Kidney

In PKD, multiple grapelike clusters of fluid-filled cysts develop in and greatly enlarge both kidneys. Eventually, dialysis or renal transplantation may be needed.

▌Renal Failure

Acute Renal Failure

The rapid deterioration of renal function with rising blood levels of urea and other nitrogenous wastes (azotemia) is termed acute renal failure (ARF). The nephrons also are unable to regulate the fluid and electrolyte or the acid-base balance of the blood.

Prerenal ARF

Any abnormal decline in kidney perfusion that reduces glomerular perfusion can cause prerenal failure.

Intrarenal ARF

Tissue damage of the glomeruli and/or tubules causes a loss of renal function known as intrarenal ARF.

Postrenal ARF

Postrenal ARF is caused by an obstruction and makes up approximately 5% of all ARF cases.

Oliguric/Nonoliguric Phase

A nonoliguric phase is usually seen when nephrotoxic agents are the causative factor. An oliguric phase, which may last 1 to 2 weeks, is seen more often when ischemia is the causative factor.

Diuretic Phase

The diuretic phase is seldom seen because early dialysis keeps extracellular fluid volume at a fairly normal level.

Recovery Phase

As renal function begins to improve, the client's urine output returns to normal and serum and urine laboratory test values move closer to normal.

Nursing Interventions

Nursing interventions for a client with acute renal failure may include the following:

1. Monitor BUN, creatinine, and serum electrolyte and protein levels.
2. Accurately measure urine output.
3. Weigh daily to identify weight gain related to fluid retention.
4. Assess skin turgor, edema, BP, lung sounds, jugular vein distention, pulse and respiratory rate and quality.
5. Provide fluids within the prescribed limits.
6. Suggest 6 small meals throughout the day.
7. Offer antinausea medications before meals.

Chronic Renal Failure (End-Stage Renal Disease)

Chronic renal failure is a slow, progressive condition in which the kidney's ability to function ultimately

deteriorates. This condition is not reversible.

Nursing Interventions

Nursing interventions for a client with ESRD may include the following:

1. Monitor daily weight, intake and output (maybe hourly), skin turgor, edema, blood pressure, respirations, and lung sounds.
2. Provide prescribed amounts of fluids.
3. Provide or assist with complete mouth care before meals because uremic halitosis leaves a metallic taste in the client's mouth.
4. Administer antiemetics 30 minutes before meals to control nausea.
5. Bathe skin frequently to remove "uremic frost."
6. Encourage the client to discuss feelings about long-term lifestyle changes.

DIALYSIS

As the kidneys continue to deteriorate, nitrogenous waste products accumulate in the circulatory system. These waste products then need to be removed artificially with dialysis. Dialysis is a mechanical means of removing nitrogenous waste from the blood by imitating the function of the nephrons.

Hemodialysis

Hemodialysis is performed by a machine with an artificial semipermeable membrane used for the filtration of the blood.

Peritoneal Dialysis

Peritoneal dialysis uses the peritoneal lining of the abdominal cavity as the membrane through which diffusion and osmosis occur instead of the artificial kidney machine. It is usually performed 4 times a day 7 days a week. A Tenckhoff or a flanged-collar catheter is placed by the physician, under aseptic conditions, into the client's peritoneal space. The client must void just before catheter insertion to prevent accidental puncture of the bladder. As with hemodialysis, the client should be weighed before and after each dialysis session. The nurse also checks bowel sounds.

The dialysate is instilled aseptically through the catheter into the abdominal cavity. To decrease client discomfort, the dialysate should be at body temperature and not instilled too rapidly.

KIDNEY TRANSPLANTATION

Transplants are either from a live donor (usually a relative) or from a cadaver.

Nursing Interventions

Nursing interventions for a client with kidney transplantation may nclude the following:

1. Monitor urine output, blood tests, vital signs, and level of consciousness.
2. Encourage turning, coughing, and deep breathing.
3. Assess the incision to ensure that wound closures are intact.
4. Assess for rejection.

Organ Rejection

Signs of rejection include generalized edema, tenderness over the graft site, fever, decreased urine output, hematuria, edema (extremities or eyes), weight gain, oliguria or anuria, and/or an increase in feeling tired. The BUN and creatinine will be elevated.

Complications

The greatest complication in renal transplantation is infection. Teach the client and family how to recognize these signs of infection: only a slight increase in temperature, development of a cough, low back pain, cloudy urine, or wound drainage. The client must always monitor urine output.

NURSING CARE OF THE CLIENT: FEMALE REPRODUCTIVE SYSTEM

CHAPTER 30

Pelvic Inflammatory Disease

Pelvic inflammatory disease (PID) is an inflammatory process involving pathogenic invasion of the fallopian tubes (salpingitis) or ovaries (oophoritis), or both, as well as any vascular or supporting structures within the pelvis, except the uterus.

Nursing Interventions

Nursing interventions for a client with pelvic inflammatory disease may include the following:

1. Assess client's pain level every 4 hours, noting the location, duration, sensation, intensity, and factors that increase or decrease the pain.
2. Explain the importance of completing the entire course of antibiotics and other medications to ensure eradication of the pathogens from the pelvic organs.
3. Encourage the client to maintain a semi-Fowler's position to prevent the spread of inflammation to pelvic organs.

Toxic Shock Syndrome

Toxic shock syndrome (TSS) is a condition most often associated with *Staphylococcus aureus,* which enters the bloodstream.

Nursing Interventions

Nursing interventions for a client with toxic shock syndrome may include the following:

1. Administer antiemetic and antidiarrheal medications as ordered. Assess skin turgor and mucous membranes.
2. Monitor I & O.

Fibroid Tumors

Fibroids (leiomyomas) are benign tumors that grow in or on the uterus.

Nursing Interventions

Nursing interventions for a client with fibroids may include the following:

1. Assess client's blood loss for amount, color, and clots.

2. Provide an accurate count of the saturated sanitary pads, along with the length of time taken to saturate a pad.
3. Monitor vital signs at least every 4 hours.

Breast Cancer

Breast cancers often occur in the upper, outer quadrant of the breast and may extend into the tail of the breast and spread upward into the axilla.

Nursing Interventions

Nursing interventions for a client with breast cancer may include the following:

1. Encourage client to express specific feelings of fear.
2. Encourage client recommended for chemotherapy to obtain a wig before therapy begins.
3. Inform client that she may have decreased sensation and lymphatic fluid retention in the arm on the affected side.
4. Teach client to keep arm on affected side elevated above the level of the heart to promote lymph drainage.
5. Assess the client's breath sounds, rate, and quality of respirations every 4 hours.
6. Monitor O_2 saturation with pulse oximeter.
7. Encourage deep breathing or the use of incentive spirometry every hour.
8. Medicate the client or encourage use of the PCA pump.

9. Encourage active ROM as soon as ordered by the physician.

Cervical Cancer

An abnormal condition of the cervix known as dysplasia may be an early sign of developing cervical cancer. Carcinoma *in situ* (CIS) means that the cancerous cells remain within the cervix and have not yet spread to adjacent areas. Stages II through IV indicate that the cancer cells have invaded the bladder, vagina, or other pelvic organs.

Nursing Interventions

Nursing interventions for a client with cervical cancer may include the following:

1. Be aware of the client's emotional state throughout the course of care and use effective interpersonal communication to facilitate the client's acceptance of her condition and the treatments.
2. Inform client that she may experience dyspareunia related to vaginal dryness after radiation therapy.
3. Instruct client to use a water-soluble lubricant during intercourse or to use lubricated condoms to decrease irritation.
4. Encourage the client to drink many fluids to flush the kidneys and decrease risk of UTI.

Endometrial Cancer

Postmenopausal women are at the greatest risk for endometrial cancer, especially if they have taken estrogen replacement therapy for several years.

Ovarian Cancer

Ovarian cancer most often originates in the epithelial tissue of the ovary, and, like cervical and endometrial cancer, does not produce symptoms until it is in an advanced, inoperable stage and is sometimes called "the silent killer."

Nursing Interventions

Nursing interventions for a client with endometrial or ovarian cancer may include the following:

1. Provide the client with proper skin care instructions during and after radiation therapy that may include avoiding soaps, creams, powder, deodorants, and other substances around the incision that may irritate the skin; not washing off the radiation markings; and avoiding tight clothing around the area.
2. Teach the client to look for signs of reactions to radiation therapy, such as tenderness, flushed color (like a sunburn), delayed wound healing, and itching.
3. Perform daily cleansing of the incisional area with water only.
4. If the client is on complete bed rest due to radium implant therapy, provide a complete bedbath as well as morning and bedtime skin care.
5. Put soiled dressings in a biohazard waste container.
6. Forewarn the client of radiation enteritis and cystitis, and common tissue responses to radiation ther-

apy. Instruct her to report symptoms, such as diarrhea, cramping, frequency, urgency, and dysuria.
7. Assess bowel sounds and abdominal distention at least every 4 to 8 hours.
8. Carefully monitor the client's urinary pattern and maintain an accurate intake and output record.
9. Observe urine and stool for color, consistency, amount, and the presence of blood.
10. Apply thigh-high antiembolitic stockings (TEDS) as ordered.
11. Assist client to ambulate when allowed.

Cystocele, Urethrocele, Rectocele, Prolapsed Uterus

A cystocele is a downward displacement of the bladder into the anterior vaginal wall. A urethrocele is a downward displacement of the urethra into the vagina, and a rectocele is an anterior displacement of the rectum into the posterior vaginal wall. Prolapsed uterus is a downward displacement of the uterus into the vagina.

Surgery for a prolapsed uterus may require a hysterectomy. If the prolapse is accompanied by a cystocele or rectocele, an A&P repair may also be performed. An A&P repair (anterior/posterior colporrhaphy) may be performed vaginally to place the bladder, urethra, or rectum in the correct anatomic position. Another procedure, the Marshall-Marchette-Krantz, may be performed to attach the bladder to the inferior surface of the pubic bone. Postoperatively, the client may be sent home with an indwelling Foley catheter because of the potential inability to void.

Nursing Interventions

Nursing interventions for a female client with a cystocele, urethrocele, rectocele, or prolapsed uterus may include the following:

1. Teach the client Kegel exercises and encourage routine practice daily.

2. Encourage client to empty bladder frequently.
3. Encourage client to defecate at same time each day.
4. Encourage regular exercise.
5. Encourage client to eat high-fiber foods and to drink plenty of fluids.
6. Be sensitive to client cues related to her sexual concerns.

NURSING CARE OF THE CLIENT: MALE REPRODUCTIVE SYSTEM

Benign Prostatic Hyperplasia

Benign prostatic hyperplasia (BPH) is a progressive adenomatous enlargement of the prostate gland that occurs with aging.

Nursing Interventions

Nursing interventions for a postoperative client having a TURP for benign prostatic hyperplasia may include the following:

1. Maintain traction on the urethral catheter by anchoring the catheter to the leg with tape, taking care that accidental additional traction will not occur with leg movement.
2. Monitor for signs of bladder spasm pain.
3. Accurately record I&O including irrigation fluid.
4. Monitor for changes in the client's behavior, especially confusion and agitation, which may be the first signs of cerebral edema.
5. Monitor for hypertension, bradycardia, weakness, and seizures.
6. Advise the client that temporary urinary incontinence frequently occurs after surgery, and reassure him that this is normal.
7. Teach the client perineal exercises that will help him regain urinary control. These exercises consist of tightening and relaxing gluteal muscles and are to be used each time the client urinates.
8. Encourage the client to maintain a fluid intake of 2,500 to 3,000 mL/day.
9. Teach the client that vigorous exercise, driving, stair climbing, sexual activity, and lifting more than 10 pounds should be avoided until approved by the physician.
10. Instruct the client to avoid straining at stool and to use stool softeners or mild cathartics as ordered.
11. Instruct the client to report any bleeding or diminished urinary stream to the physician.
12. Monitor the client's statements to determine if he has any misunderstanding of the surgery and sexual function.
13. Advise the client that it is normal and not harmful if his urine has a milky appearance due to retrograde ejaculation.

14. Increase rate of flow of the bladder irrigant if the urine has clots, a darker color, or decreased output.

Prostate Cancer

Most prostatic cancers are adenocarcinomas, slow-growing tumors that spread through the lymphatics.

Nursing Interventions

Nursing interventions for a client (postoperative) with prostate cancer may include the following:

1. Monitor the client's urinary output, noting the amount, color, and presence of clots.
2. Reposition or milk the catheter tubing if not patent. If these interventions fail, notify the physician.
3. Monitor the client's intake, encouraging a fluid intake of 2,500 to 3,000 mL/day.
4. Advise the client that temporary urinary incontinence frequently occurs following surgery, and reassure him that this is normal.
5. Teach the client perineal exercises that will help him regain urinary control. These exercises consist of tightening and relaxing perineal (Kegel exercises) and gluteal muscles and can be performed in a variety of ways.
6. Advise the client that temporary fecal incontinence frequently occurs after a perineal incision.
7. Teach the client perineal exercises that will help him regain bowel control.

8. Avoid the use of rectal thermometers, rectal examinations, and enemas.
9. Keep the client clean and dry, especially if he is experiencing fecal or urinary incontinence.
10. Reposition client every 2 hours.

Testicular Cancer

The etiology is unknown, but the incidence is highest in men with undescended testicles and those whose mothers had taken hormones during pregnancy. A small, hard, painless lump is usually the first symptom noted.

Nursing Interventions

Nursing interventions for the client with testicular cancer may include the following:

1. Monitor the client's vital signs and incisional drainage.
2. Report hyperthermia, tachycardia, hypotension, increased incisional drainage, and swelling or redness around the incision to the physician immediately.
3. Maintain strict asepsis when handling wound dressings.
4. Provide the client with opportunities to voice concerns and ask questions.
5. Advise the client that he needs to be on bed rest for 12 to 24 hours postoperatively.
6. Instruct the client to wear tight-fitting underwear or an athletic supporter when ambulating and to avoid heavy lifting for 4 to 6 weeks.

Penile Cancer

Penile cancer is rare and has a high correlation with poor hygiene and delayed or no circumcision.

Nursing Interventions

Nursing interventions for a client with penile cancer may include the following:

1. Monitor the client's vital signs and incisional drainage.
2. Report hyperthermia, tachycardia, hypotension, increased incisional drainage, and swelling or redness around the incision to the physician immediately.
3. Maintain strict asepsis when handling wound dressings.
4. Report low urinary output to the physician immediately.

Structural Disorders

Cryptorchidism is a condition in which one or both testicles fail to descend into the scrotum by the time of birth.

A hydrocele is a benign, nontender collection of clear, amber fluid within the space of the testes and the tunica vaginalis or along the spermatic cord.

Hypospadias is an abnormal placement of the urethral opening on the ventral surface of the penis. Epispadias is the opening of the urethra on the dorsal surface of the penis.

A spermatocele is a benign nontender cyst of either the epididymis or the rete testis. It contains milky fluid and sperm.

A varicocele is dilation of the veins of the scrotum that occurs when the venous system that drains the testicle lengthens and enlarges.

Torsion of the spermatic cord occurs when the vascular pedicle of the testis twists, resulting in partial or complete venous occlusion.

NURSING CARE OF THE CLIENT: SEXUALLY TRANSMITTED DISEASES

Common sexually-transmitted diseases are discussed in Table 32-1.

Table 32–1 SEXUALLY TRANSMITTED DISEASES: AN OVERVIEW

DISEASE	CHARACTERISTICS
Chlamydia	*Male:* Painful urination Urethral discharge *Female:* Asymptomatic or may experience purulent discharge *Note:* If untreated, pelvic inflammatory disease (PID) can develop.
Cytomegalo-virus (CMV)	Often asymptomatic, occasionally fever, fatigue, and weakness Generally acquired during childhood or adolescence 80% to 100% of adults have antibodies to CMV.
Genital Herpes: Herpes Simplex Virus 2 (HSV-2)	Vesicles on penis, vagina, labia, perineum, or anus Can progress to painful ulceration Lasts up to 6 weeks Recurrence common *Note:* May be asymptomatic
Gonorrhea	*Male:* Urethritis (inflammation of the urethra) Purulent discharge Urinary frequency Epididymitis (inflammation of the epididymis) *Female:* Often asymptomatic May lead to PID or salpingitis (inflammation of the fallopian tube) Can occlude the fallopian tubes, resulting in sterility

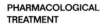

PHARMACOLOGICAL TREATMENT	NURSING IMPLICATIONS
Vibramycin is the treatment of choice. Zithromax can be given orally in a single dose. Ilosone or Amoxil is given to pregnant women but they should be cultured again after treatment is completed to confirm the absence of disease.	Instruct client to notify sexual partner(s) of past 2 months of their need for treatment. Instruct client to avoid sexual activity or to use condoms until both client and partner(s) are symptom free. Provide instruction regarding medications prescribed.
There is no antiviral agent specifically utilized for this disorder, since most of the population will not have any symptoms.	Implicated in some spontaneous abortions or mental retardation. Congenital infection produces cytomegalic inclusion disease. May be life threatening in a client with a poorly functioning immune system.
A topical form of Zovirax may be applied to the lesions or the drug may also be taken orally to shorten the duration of the lesions in a primary outbreak. When taken daily, it prevents most recurrences. Famivir and Valtrex suppress viral activity and also prevent recurrences.	Refer sexual partner(s) for examination. Teach that virus can be transmitted even when the person experiences no symptoms. Instruct in use of condoms. Teach females of need for annual Pap smear. Provide instruction regarding medications prescribed.
One of the most effective therapies is a single dose of Cipro followed by a 7-day course of oral Vibramycin. A pregnant client or a client under 16 is given an injection of Rocephlin followed by oral Ilosone.	Instruct client to return if symptoms persist. Sexual partner(s) of past 60 days must be assessed Instruct client to avoid sexual activity until symptoms subside in both client and partner(s). Provide instruction regarding medications prescribed.

(continues)

DISEASE	CHARACTERISTICS
Hepatitis B Virus (HBV)	Varies greatly from asymptomatic state to severe hepatitis to cancer
Genital Warts (Human Papilloma-virus)	Fleshy, cauliflowerlike growth on genitalia
Syphilis	Disease consists of 4 stages with distinct manifestations as follows:
	Primary:
	A painless papule on penis, vagina, or cervix (chancre)
	Usually negative serologic blood test
	Highly infectious during this stage
	Secondary:
	Rash, especially prevalent on palms and soles
	Low-grade fever
	Sore throat
	Headache
	Early latency:
	Possible infectious lesions, otherwise asymptomatic
	Reactive serologic tests

PHARMACOLOGICAL TREATMENT	NURSING IMPLICATIONS
There is no specific therapy. Treatment is based on relieving symptoms.	Partner(s) should receive medical prophylaxis within 14 days after exposure. For client and partner(s), recommend three-dose immunization series when this episode has abated.
A topical solution of Poddoen may be applied to the genital warts. It is only recommended for treatment of 1 or 2 lesions at a time, since it can be toxic if applied to too large an area at one time. After the solution has been in contact with the genital warts for a period of 4 to 6 hours, it is then washed off with soap and water. If not thoroughly washed off, Poddoen may cause chemical burns that heal very slowly and are very painful. A cream, Aldara is applied before bedtime and washed off in the morning. It can be used 3 times a week for 16 weeks or less.	Inform and treat sexual partner(s). Provide instruction regarding medications prescribed.
Bicillin L-A is often the preferred penicillin. If the client has a demonstrated allergy to penicillin, alternative medications are Vibramycin, Achromycin V, or Ilosone. Pregnant women who are allergic to penicillin are given erythromycin.	Interview client to identify sexual contacts. All those exposed to the disease should be given penicillin. Educate client and sexual contacts about the disease. Provide instruction regarding medications prescribed. Counsel and educate client.

(*continues*)

Table 32–1 (continued)

DISEASE	CHARACTERISTICS
Syphilis (continued)	*Late latency:*
	Possible lesions in central nervous and cardiovascular systems
	Noninfectious except to fetus of pregnant woman
Trichomoniasis	Petechial lesions
	Profuse urethral or vaginal discharge that is foul smelling, yellow, and foamy

PHARMACOLOGICAL TREATMENT	NURSING IMPLICATIONS
	Counsel and educate client.
Both partners should be treated with Flagyl either given orally in a singled dose or for a period of approximately 1 week. If given vaginally, Flagyl is not as effective.	Treat sexual partners simultaneously with metronidazole (Flagyl). Provide instruction regarding medication prescribed.

NURSING CARE OF THE CLIENT: MENTAL ILLNESS

THE CLIENT EXPERIENCING A CRISIS

In psychological terms, a crisis is a stressor that forces an individual to respond and/or adapt in some way.

The Client Is Anxious

Anxiety is a state wherein a person feels a strong sense of dread frequently accompanied by physical symptoms of increased heart and respiratory rates and elevated blood pressure in the absence of a specific source or reason for these emotions or responses (Table 33–1).

Generalized Anxiety Disorder

The client with generalized anxiety disorder (GAD) exhibits symptoms of excessive anxiety or dread.

Panic Disorder

Panic disorder is a condition wherein the client experiences periods of intense anxiety that begin abruptly and peak within 10 minutes.

Post-traumatic Stress Disorder

Clients suffering from post-traumatic stress disorder (PTSD) have experienced a serious trauma. The response to the trauma must have been one of fear or helplessness, and the event is persistently re-experienced through recurrent recollections, dreams, or hallucinatory-like flashbacks.

Nursing Interventions

Nursing interventions for the client with anxiety may include the following:

1. Teach the client relaxation exercises.
2. Explore with the client those things that are calming and relaxing.
3. Encourage physical movement or participation in some type of recreational or sporting activity to release excess energy.
4. Remain with the client while level of fear is high.
5. Talk to the client in a calm, soothing voice.

Table 33-1 ASKING CLIENTS ABOUT SYMPTOMS OF ANXIETY DISORDERS

Following are questions that have proven useful in eliciting information from clients about symptoms of anxiety disorders. You may find that you prefer to word these questions somewhat differently, but the important thing is to ask them. Many clients experience anxiety symptoms for years before a doctor, nurse, or psychologist takes the time to ask about these symptoms.

Generalized anxiety disorder	Do you find yourself worrying frequently about a number of different things, such as the way things are going for you at home, work, or school?
	Do you find yourself feeling anxious or tense much of the time without any obvious reason?
Panic disorder	Have you ever experienced sudden, intense fear for no reason?
	Have you found yourself experiencing intense physical symptoms of chest pain, shortness of breath, dizziness, or sweating, along with a sense that something terrible or life threatening was happening to you?
Post-traumatic stress disorder	Have you ever had a particularly traumatic experience such as witnessing or experiencing violence or a catastrophic event (such as a flood or fire)?
	Have you ever found yourself reexperiencing a violent or catastrophic event through dreams or waking "flashbacks"?

From *Psychiatric Mental Health Nursing*, 2nd ed., *by N. Frisch and L. Frisch, 2002, Albany, NY: Delmar. Copyright 2002 by Delmar.*

6. Reassure the client that he is in a safe place.
7. Orient the client to reality, if the client is confused, disoriented, or experiencing flashbacks.

The Client Who Is Depressed

Depression is the state wherein an individual experiences feelings of extreme sadness, hopelessness, and helplessness.

Major Depressive Disorder

To qualify for the diagnosis of Major Depressive Disorder, DSM-IV requires the presence of at least one Major Depressive Episode. This episode must (1) last at least 2 weeks, (2) represent a change from previous functioning, and (3) cause some impairment in a person's social or occupational functioning.

Dysthymic Disorder

Persons with Dysthymic Disorder feel depressed nearly all of the time.

Nursing Interventions

Nursing interventions for the client with depression may include the following:

1. Build rapport and develop therapeutic relationship with client.
2. Spend time with client individually.
   Encourage client to interact with others.
3. Encourage client to initiate conversation with others.
4. Verbally praise client for increasing interactions and initiating conversation.
5. Praise client for each activity done on own.

THE CLIENT WHO IS POTENTIALLY VIOLENT

Homicidal

The client who is homicidal is planning or threatening to harm or kill another individual or individuals.

Suicidal

Clients who are suicidal often feel overwhelmed by life events and decide that the only relief will come from ending their own lives. Assessment of risk for suicide is shown in Table 33–2.

Table 33–2 ASSESSMENT OF RISK FOR SUICIDE

The following areas are to be assessed in all potentially suicidal clients:

1. Does the client have a *plan* to commit suicide?

Example: Client plans to "end it all" after wife leaves for work on a Monday.

Rationale: Some clients may be experiencing thoughts of wishing they were dead or killing themselves, but may not have a plan for doing so. *The client who has a plan for committing suicide is at increased risk.*

2. How *specific* is the plan to commit suicide?

Example: Client states he plans to overdose on sleeping pills.

Rationale: A specific plan increases the risk of completing a suicide.

3. Does the client have access to the *means* to commit suicide?

Example: Client states he will use his spouse's sleeping pills to overdose.

Rationale: Easy availability of the means to kill oneself increases the risk of suicide.

4. How *lethal* is the intended means to commit suicide?

Example: Client states he will "blow his brains out" with a gun.

Rationale: Some means of suicide are more likely to result in a completed suicide. *Gunshots are the most common cause of completed suicide.* The lethality of guns makes the potential for a successful intervention very slim. Intervention in light of means that are less lethal may yield a more favorable outcome (e.g., overdose, cutting of wrists).

Nursing Interventions

Nursing interventions for the client who is severely agitated, aggressive, actively suicidal, and/or homicidal may include the following:

1. Assess for the presence of suicidal thoughts and whether a specific plan is present.
2. Evaluate the degree of risk associated with the client's verbalization of suicide intent.
3. Contact the attending physician or psychiatrist and inform of the client's intentions and current condition (Isaacs, 1998).
4. Assess and evaluate the client's surroundings and environment for any potentially dangerous items or objects that could be used for self-harm.
5. Remove or secure any potentially harmful items after thoroughly evaluating the situation.
6. Increase the level of observation so that the client is frequently monitored.
7. Assist the client in developing a No-suicide Contract (Badger, 1995).
8. Assess for the presence of homicidal ideations.
9. If the client is verbalizing a plan to harm someone, immediately notify the proper authorities so they can alert this individual.

THE CLIENT WHO IS PSYCHOTIC

Psychosis is a state wherein an individual loses the ability to recognize reality.

Schizophrenia

Clients with schizophrenia frequently have belief systems that have become distorted in some manner, so that they hold firmly to false ideas or delusions, even when presented with evidence to the contrary.

Family involvement is important for all clients, but it is especially critical for the client with schizophrenia. Because the client may be too ill or confused to be trusted to take medications reliably, it becomes the responsibility of family members to help ensure medication compliance.

Nursing Interventions

Nursing interventions for the client with schizophrenia may include the following:

1. Assess for the presence of hallucinations.
2. Assist the client in beginning to exert some control over the hallucinations.
3. Educate the client about ways to decrease the intensity and power of the hallucinations.
4. Educate the client and family about the disorder of schizophrenia.
5. Educate the client and family about the need for antipsychotic medications.
6. Educate the client and family about the importance of continuing the prescribed medication regimen.

The Client with Bipolar Disorder

Bipolar Disorder (previously known as manic–depressive disorder) is a psychiatric diagnosis characterized by wide fluctuations in mood (the way an individual reports feeling, e.g., depressed, elated, happy, sad) and affect (the objective or outward manifestation of the way an individual is feeling, e.g., avoids eye contact, smiles occasionally). In addition to having a wide range of both affect and mood, the individual with bipolar disorder may experience fluctuations between depression and mania (extremely elevated mood with accompanying agitated behavior).

Nursing Interventions

Nursing interventions for the client with bipolar disorder may include the following:

1. Provide a quiet, peaceful environment.
2. Teach client relaxation exercises.
3. Educate the client and family about the disease process and the progression of the illness over time.
4. Educate the client and family about prescribed medication, indications for use, dosage, times, and any possible side effects or untoward reactions.
5. Educate the client and family about the importance of taking the medication as prescribed.
6. Teach the client to continue taking medication and to not miss doses *even if the condition improves dramatically.*

The Client Experiencing Neglect and/or Abuse

There are many types of neglect (a situation wherein a basic need of the client is not being provided) and abuse (an incident involving some type of violation to the client).

Elder Abuse and Neglect

The House Select Committee on Aging defined the following types of elder abuse: physical, passive physical, financial, psychological, sexual, and violation of rights.

Domestic Violence

Domestic violence occurs in relationships in which intentional or controlling behavior is perpetrated by persons with whom a survivor has had or currently has an intimate relationship. The syndrome may include actual or threatened physical injury, sexual assault, psychological abuse, economic control, and/or progressive isolation. (Medical Education Group Learning Systems, 1995).

Rape

Rape is a legal term, not a medical entity. It is a crime of violence. Rapists use sexual violence to dominate and degrade their victims and to express their own anger. It is not an act of lust or an overzealous release of passion done to satisfy a sexual urge (Frisch & Frisch 2002).

Nursing Interventions

Nursing interventions for the client experiencing neglect or abuse may include the following:

1. Document the evidence of neglect with which the client presents via written observations, laboratory reports, and/or pictures, if indicated.
2. Report the case of neglect to the proper authorities: police, child protective services (CPS), APS, and any others that might be indicated.
3. Reassure the client that the client is in a safe place and that you are there to help in any way that you can.

Eating Disorders

Anorexia nervosa is characterized by self-imposed starvation by restricting caloric intake and compulsive exercising. Bulimia nervosa is characterized by periods of binge eating of up to 10,000 calories at one time followed by self-induced vomiting and other forms of purging such as laxative and diuretic abuse.

Nursing Interventions

Nursing interventions for a hospitalized client with anorexia nervosa or bulimia nervosa may include the following:

1. Weigh daily.
2. Monitor calorie intake.
3. Administer IV rehydration, electrolyte replacement, and TPN or tube feedings as ordered.
4. Monitor behavior at and around meal time, such as going to the bathroom right after eating.
5. Monitor exercise patterns.
6. Monitor I & O every shift and bowel movements for diarrhea (a sign of continued laxative abuse).

REFERENCES

Badger, J. (1995). Reaching out to the suicidal patient. *American Journal of Nursing, 95*(30), 24–31.

Frisch, N. C. & Frisch, L. E. (2002). *Psychiatric mental health nursing*. Albany, NY: Delmar.

Isaacs, A. (1998). Depression and your patient. *American Journal of Nursing, 98*(7), 26–31.

Medical Education Group Learning Systems. (1995). *Domestic violence: A practical guide for physicians* [On-line]. Available: http://www.cme.edu/phydom/domes.html

NURSING CARE OF THE CLIENT: SUBSTANCE ABUSE

CHAPTER 34

CNS Depressants

Substances in this category include alcohol, benzodiazepines, and cannabis.

Alcohol

Low doses of alcohol depress areas of the brain that are inhibitory, causing diminished self-control and impaired judgment. Continued alcohol ingestion may cause unconsciousness and even death.

Treatment/Rehabilitation

Many treatment programs are based in hospital or residential treatment centers. These are generally called inpatient programs and last 30 days.

Education

The abuse of or dependence on alcohol is a maladaptive way to cope with life stressors. Learning basic life skills to improve personal competence and provide adaptive coping mechanisms helps the individual resist the use of alcohol.

Self-Help Groups

Alcoholics Anonymous (AA) is the model for other self-help groups such as AL-ANON for adults, AL-ATEEN for teenage children, and AL-ATOT for younger children in the family of an alcoholic.

Benzodiazepines and Other Sedative-Hypnotics

Incidence

Benzodiazepines are not commonly used as recreational drugs but are widely prescribed and are thus available for abuse.

Treatment/Rehabilitation

Ideally, treatment for benzodiazepine abuse is a gradual reduction in the amount taken until the client is no longer taking any. A cross-tolerant drug such as phenobarbital is sometimes given to control symptoms and then its dosage is reduced. Hospital treatment is likely to be needed.

Cannabis

Marijuana is the most common type of cannabis used.

Treatment/Rehabilitation

Treatment focuses on relapse prevention and the development of new coping mechanisms, ways of living, and means of having fun without drugs. Weekly group therapy sessions to maintain a commitment to abstinence and enhance interpersonal skills are often used. Participation in a self-help group is encouraged.

CNS Stimulants

Substances in this category include cocaine and amphetamines.

Cocaine

Cocaine is extracted from the leaves of the coca plant, *Erythroxylum coca*. It may be heated and the fumes inhaled. This is termed *freebasing*. As a white powder, cocaine may be snorted by inhaling it through the nose. It may also be heated to a liquid state and injected intravenously. Crack is a crystallized form of cocaine that is melted in a water pipe and smoked.

Treatment/Rehabilitation

Treatment is aimed at reducing the craving and managing the severe depression. Careful monitoring of the client is necessary to identify and prevent actions aimed at carrying out the idea of suicide. Inpatient programs for some clients with cocaine dependence should therefore be recommended, while other clients can be effectively treated in outpatient programs.

Amphetamines

Amphetamines (also called uppers, speed, bennies) include dextroamphetamine sulfate (Dexedrine), amphetamine sulfate (Amphetamine), and methamphetamine hydrochloride (Desoxyn). Medically they are used to treat attention deficit hyperactivity disorder (ADHD), narcolepsy, and obesity.

Treatment/Rehabilitation

Urinary acidifiers, such as ascorbic acid (vitamin C), increase the excretion of amphetamines. Diazepam (Valium) is given for sedation to ease the withdrawal crash. Bromocriptine mesylate (Parlodel) or levodopa (Dopar) may help decrease the craving. A quiet environment is also helpful.

Behavioral therapy is used to help the client recognize and accept the need to stop using amphetamines. Supportive individual or group therapy, and especially self-help groups, aids the client to stay abstinent and in treatment.

Hallucinogens

Hallucinogens refers to a group of naturally occurring and synthetic agents that produce essentially the same mind-altering effects.

Lysergic Acid Diethylamide

Lysergic acid diethylamide (LSD), a manufactured chemical compound, is perhaps the most widely known and used hallucinogen.

Treatment/Rehabilitation

A person on a "bad trip" should be carefully watched to prevent self-injury. Reassurance, support, and "talking down" should be done in a quiet, pleasant manner. The person should be encouraged to sit up or walk. Closing the eyes intensifies the "bad trip." The person should be reminded that the drug is causing the effects, which will soon go away.

After cessation of chronic LSD use, long-term psychotherapy is usually required to determine what needs were fulfilled by the use of this drug. A 12-step program and family assistance are usually necessary to reinforce the decision to remain abstinent. If the client is upset by flashbacks or the fear of flashbacks, an anxiolytic drug such as diazepam (Valium) may be ordered.

Phencyclidine

Phencyclidine (PCP) was made for use as an anesthetic agent, but it produced such adverse reactions that it was withdrawn from clinical trials.

Treatment/Rehabilitation

Treatment should begin in an inpatient setting because of the high risk of suicide. Sedatives may be used and urinary acidifiers such as ascorbic acid may be given to increase excretion of PCP. No effort should be made to "talk down" or calm the individual. Diazepam (Valium) may be ordered.

Body awareness, yoga, and progressive relaxation help the client focus and improve attention span and concentration. Participation in a self-help group such as Narcotics Anonymous (NA) should be encouraged, though initial involvement is usually minimal.

Opioids

Opioids is a term used to refer to naturally occurring opiates, semisynthetic opiates, synthetic opiates, and agonist-antagonists.

Treatment/Rehabilitation

Initial treatment is symptomatic and supportive of vital functions until the acute phase is over.

Detoxification

Several methods currently used for opioid detoxification are methadone, LAAM, and naltrexone. Individual and/or group counseling must go hand in hand with the detoxification to help the client learn new methods of coping with life's stresses.

NURSING CARE OF THE OLDER CLIENT

Aging (senescence) is a complex phenomenon that occurs on the continuum of human life, beginning with birth and continuing throughout the lifespan, and to the end stages of life and death.

The clinical delineation of an older adult is still someone who is 65 years of age or older; older-old adults are defined as those individuals 85 years of age or older.

The battle continues against the stereotyping of older adults, both in the health professions and in the community at large. Health professionals, in particular, must be diligent in avoiding age prejudice, as believing stereotypes can influence interactions between older adults and caregivers.

Aging is universal, progressive, and irreversible and eventually leads to death. The aging process itself, however, is very individualized and is independent of chronological age.

HEALTH AND AGING

Adaptive devices and techniques are available for those who need assistance with the activities of daily living (ADLs), basic care activities that include mobility, bathing, hygiene, grooming, and dressing.

Mobility

Handrails can decrease the risk of falls while the person is walking; they are also useful in the tub and, when used in conjunction with a plastic riser, can help the older adult get on and off the toilet safely.

Bathing

Skin dryness increases with aging; thus, it may be preferable for older adults to bathe or shower only two to three times per week and to take sponge baths in between.

Hygiene

Fingernails may become more brittle with aging. Impaired circulation is common among older adults, and special attention should thus be given to care of the feet and lower extremities.

Grooming

Good grooming is important in promoting the older client's self-esteem and confidence.

Dressing

Many choices are available to ease dressing, such as elastic waists, velcro fasteners, and assistive reaching and dressing devices.

Eating

Dysphagia, or difficulty swallowing, may place the older client at increased risk of choking, and diminished taste sensation may affect the desire to eat.

Toileting

It is extremely important that caregivers of older adults monitor bowel patterns. Long periods of constipation (> than 2 to 3 days) should alert caregivers to the need for interventions to minimize the likelihood of bowel impaction, which can ultimately be life threatening if left untreated. Evacuation aids such as laxatives, lubricants, stool softeners, and enemas all have side-effects and should thus be avoided if at all possible. Dietary changes or an exercise regimen should be introduced first.

EXERCISE

What was once accepted as the normal deterioration of old age is now considered the result of disuse through sitting and bed rest. Research indicates that high-intensity, progressive resistance training can improve muscle strength and muscle size in frail elderly clients.

NUTRITION

There are no universally accepted dietary guidelines specific to older adults.

PSYCHOSOCIAL CONSIDERATIONS

Mental activity and emotional involvement are as necessary to the overall well-being as is physical activity.

PHYSIOLOGIC CHANGES ASSOCIATED WITH AGING

Although the aging process brings with it many physiologic changes, it should be remembered that aging and disease are not synonymous. The physiologic changes of aging described following are normal for most people.

Respiratory System

- The muscles of respiration become less flexible, causing decreased vital capacity of the lungs.
- Decrease in functional capacity results in dyspnea on exertion or stress; usual activity does not affect breathing.
- Effectiveness of the cough mechanism lessens, increasing the risk of lung infection.
- The alveoli thicken and decrease in number and size, causing less effective gas exchange.
- Structural changes in the skeleton, such as kyphosis (seen in clients

with osteoporosis as an often asymetrical convex curve of the spine) can decrease diaphragmatic expansion.

Cardiovascular System

- Cardiac output and recovery time decline.
- The heart rate slows.
- Blood flow to all organs decreases.
- Arterial elasticity decreases, causing increased peripheral resistance and, in turn, a rise in systolic blood pressure and a slight rise in diastolic blood pressure.
- Veins dilate, and superficial vessels become more prominent.

Gastrointestinal System

- Tooth enamel thins.
- Periodontal disease rate increases.
- Taste buds decrease in number, and saliva production diminishes.
- Effectiveness of the gag reflex lessens, resulting in an increased risk of choking.
- Esophageal peristalsis slows, and the effectiveness of the esophageal sphincter lessens, causing delayed entry of food into the stomach and increasing the risk of aspiration.
- Hiatal hernia may occur.
- Gastric emptying slows.
- Peristalsis and nerve sensation of the large intestine decreases, contributing to constipation.
- The incidence of diverticulosis increases with age.
- Liver size decreases after age 70.
- Liver enzymes decrease, slowing drug metabolism and the detoxification process.
- Emptying of the gallbladder lessens

in efficiency, resulting in thickened bile, increased cholesterol content, and increased incidence of gallstones.

Reproductive System: Female

- Estrogen production decreases with the onset of menopause.
- Ovaries, uterus, and cervix decrease in size.
- The vagina shortens, narrows, and becomes less elastic, and the vaginal lining thins. Secretions decrease and become more alkaline, resulting in increased incidence of atrophic vaginitis.
- Supporting musculature of the reproductive organs weakens, increasing the risk of uterine prolapse.
- Breast tissue diminishes, and nipple erection lessens during sexual arousal.
- Libido and the need for intimacy and companionship in older women remain unchanged.

Reproductive System: Male

- Testosterone production decreases, resulting in decreased size of the testicles.
- Sperm count and viscosity of seminal fluid decrease.
- More time is required to obtain erection.
- The prostate gland may enlarge.
- Impotency may occur.
- Libido and the need for intimacy and companionship remain unchanged in older males.

Endocrine System

- Alterations occur in both the reception and the production of hormones.
- Release of insulin by the beta cells of the pancreas slows, causing an increase in blood sugar.
- Thyroid changes may lower the basal metabolic rate.

Musculoskeletal System

- Muscle mass and elasticity diminish, resulting in decreased strength, endurance, coordination, and increased reaction time.
- Bone demineralization occurs, causing skeletal instability and shrinkage of intervertebral disks. The flexibility of the spine lessens, and spinal curvature often occurs.
- Joints undergo degenerative changes, resulting in pain, stiffness, and loss of range of motion.

Integumentary System

- Subcutaneous tissue and elastin fibers diminish, causing the skin to become thinner and less elastic.
- Eccrine, apocrine, and sebaceous glands decrease in size, number, and function, resulting in diminished secretions and moisturization and, thus, pruritis.
- Body temperature regulation diminishes due to decreased perspiration and, many times, decreased circulation.
- Capillary blood flow decreases, resulting in slower wound healing.
- Blood flow decreases, especially to lower extremities.
- Vascular fragility causes senile purpura.

- Cutaneous sensitivity to pressure and temperature diminishes.

Neurological System

- Neurons in the brain decrease in number, resulting in decreased production of neurotransmitters and, thus, reduced synaptic transmission.
- Cerebral blood flow and oxygen utilization decrease.
- Time required to carry out motor and sensory tasks requiring speed, coordination, balance, and fine-motor hand movements increases.
- Short-term memory may somewhat diminish without much change in long-term memory.
- Night sleep disturbances occur due to more frequent and longer wakeful periods.
- Deep-tendon reflexes decrease, although reflexes at the knees remain fairly intact.

Urinary System

- Nephrons in the kidneys decrease in number and function, resulting in decreased filtration and gradual decrease in excretory and reabsorbtive functions of the renal tubules.
- Glomerular filtration rate decreases, resulting in decreased renal clearance of drugs.
- Blood urea nitrogen increases.
- Sodium-conserving ability diminishes.
- Bladder capacity decreases, causing increased frequency of urination, including nocturia.
- Renal function increases when the older client lies down, sometimes causing a need to void shortly after going to bed.

- Bladder and perineal muscles weaken, resulting in the inability to empty the bladder and predisposing the elderly client to cystitis.
- Incidence of stress incontinence increases in older females.
- The prostate may enlarge in older males, causing urinary frequency or dribbling.

NOTE: Elderly persons frequently do not present with the usual signs and symptoms of urinary tract infections (UTIs). Falling or signs of acute confusion (more than usual) may often be the major clinical manifestations.

Sensory Changes

Vision

- With aging, the lens becomes less pliable and less able to increase its curvature in order to focus on near objects, causing presbyopia (trouble seeing objects up close) and decreased accommodation. The lens also yellows, causing distorted color perceptions, with greens and blues washing out and warm colors such as reds and oranges becoming more distinct. The incidence of cataracts also increases.

- Accommodation of pupil size decreases, resulting in both decreased adjustment to changes in lighting and decreased ability to tolerate glare.
- Vitreous humor changes in consistency, causing blurred vision. Changes in the anterior chamber may increase the pressure of the aqueous humor, resulting in glaucoma.
- Lacrimal glands secrete less fluids, causing dryness and itching.

Hearing

- As aging occurs, the pinna becomes less flexible, the hair cells in the inner ear stiffen and atrophy, and cerumen (earwax) increases.
- The number of neurons in the cochlea decrease, and the blood supply lessens, causing the cochlea and the ossicles to degenerate.
- Presbycusis, the impairment of hearing in older adults, is often accompanied by a loss of tone discrimination. High-frequency tones are lost first; thus, keeping the voice low and calm and decreasing any background noise can improve the client's comprehension of the caregiver's message.

REHABILITATION, HOME HEALTH, LONG-TERM CARE, AND HOSPICE

There has been a strong emergence in the past decade of nonacute health care services. A vast increase in rehabilitation, home health, long-term care, and hospice services is evident.

REHABILITATION

Rehabilitation is a process designed to help individuals reach their optimal level of physical, mental, and psychosocial functioning. This goal is accomplished by preventing complications, modifying the effects of the disability, and increasing independence. By so doing, the individual's self-esteem is maximized, thus increasing quality of life.

HOME HEALTH CARE

Home health care encompasses many services delivered to persons in their homes and is the fastest growing segment of health care delivery. In addition to nursing personnel, various therapists and social workers may provide services on an intermittent basis.

LONG-TERM CARE

Long-term care refers to a spectrum of services provided to individuals who have an ongoing need for health care. It has traditionally meant a community-based nursing home licensed for skilled or intermediate care.

Subacute Care

Subacute care is a concept designed to provide services for clients who are out of the acute stage of their illnesses but who still require skilled nursing, monitoring, and ongoing treatments. The clients are not critically ill but do have complex medical needs. Subacute care is intended to fill the gap between the acute care hospital and the traditional long-term care facility (AHCA, 2000).

Continuing Care Retirement Communities

Continuing Care Retirement Communities (CCRC) are designed to provide continuing levels of care as the individual's health care needs change.

Assisted Living

Assisted living combines housing and services for persons who require assistance with activities of daily living. Nursing care is not provided. These are persons who cannot live alone but who do not need 24-hour care. It is a less restrictive environment than a long-term care facility and maintains the individual's independence and freedom of choice.

Adult Day Care

Adult day care provides a variety of services in a protective setting for adults who are unable to stay alone but who do not need 24-hour care.

Respite Care

Respite care may be offered by adult day care centers, long-term care facilities, or in private homes. It is intended to provide a break to caregivers and may be utilized a few hours a week, for an occasional weekend, or for longer vacations.

Foster Care

Some states are investigating the use of foster homes for individuals who cannot live independently but who do not require the services of a health care facility. The legal structure is similar to the foster home concept for children.

Role of the LP/VN

There are many more career opportunities available for the LP/VN in long-term care facilities. The nurse needs sharp assessment skills and a sound ability to make nursing judgments based on assessment findings. The nurse may wish to seek additional course work to acquire supervisory skills. LP/VNs may take the Certification Examination for Practical and Vocational Nurses in Long-Term Care (CEPN-LTC™) given by the National Council of State Boards of Nursing (NCSBN). Those who pass the examination are certified in long-term care and may use the initials "CLTC" to signify their certification.

HOSPICE

Hospice is humane, compassionate care provided to clients who can no longer benefit from curative treatment and have 6 months or less to live. The special care is designed to provide sensitivity and support, allowing clients to carry on an alert, pain-free life with other symptoms managed so the last days are spent with dignity and quality of life at home or in a homelike setting. Hospice care may be implemented in a variety of settings: the client's home, a special area of hospitals or nursing homes, or freestanding inpatient facilities. Most clients receive care at home.

REFERENCES

American Health Care Association (AHCA). (2000). Nursing facility subacute care: The quality and cost-effective alternative to hospital care. [On-line] Available: www.ahca.org/who/pubsubac.htm

NURSING CARE OF THE CLIENT: RESPONDING TO EMERGENCIES

Shock

Shock is a condition of profound hemodynamic and metabolic disturbance characterized by inadequate tissue perfusion and inadequate circulation to the vital organs (Table 37–1).

Nursing Interventions

Nursing interventions for a client in shock may include the following:

1. Initiate and maintain fluid replacement with two large-bore IV access lines.
2. Administer blood as ordered.

Table 37–1 TYPES OF SHOCK

TYPE	CAUSES
Hypovolemic	Hemorrhage*, burns
Cardiogenic	Myocardial infarction*
Toxic	Overwhelming infection
Anaphylactic	Medications*, insect bites or stings, foods
Neurogenic	Spinal cord injury

*Most common cause

3. Assess vital signs at least every 30 minutes.
4. Administer oxygen per physician order.
5. Explain all interventions as they occur, to decrease acute anxiety.
6. Allow client and family to express their fears and worries about the situation.

CARDIOPULMONARY EMERGENCIES

Cardiopulmonary emergencies are those emergencies that jeopardize the function of the heart and lungs. Many clients will suffer other related injuries associated with drowning, such as head and spinal cord injuries (Table 37–2).

Nursing Interventions

Nursing interventions for a client with a cardiopulmonary emergency may include the following:

1. Initiate CPR, if indicated.
2. Keep client medicated to alleviate painful respirations.
3. Maintain airway and breathing with suctioning, if secretions accumulate.
4. Turn client frequently to mobilize secretions.
5. Encourage deep breathing and coughing.
6. Listen to lungs hourly or more frequently to evaluate secretions and suctioning.

SIGNS AND SYMPTOMS	EMERGENCY CARE
Increased heart rate; hypotension; cold, clammy skin; profound thirst	Replace fluids
Increased heart rate; hypotension; cold, clammy skin	Initiate drug therapy for myocardial infarction; replace fluids; consider possible emergency coronary bypass surgery
Hot, dry, flushed skin; hypotension; increased heart rate	Locate source of infection and treat with broad-spectrum antibiotic; replace fluids
Throat edema in conjunction with increasing difficulty breathing; hypotension; increased heart rate	Manage ABCs; administer epinephrine (Adrenalin); administer diphenhydramine hydrochloride (Benadryl)
Slowed heart rate; hypotension	Replace fluids, administer drugs to increase blood pressure and heart rate

Table 37–2 FRESH-WATER VERSUS SALT-WATER NEAR-DROWNING

TYPE	CLIENT SYMPTOMS	PATHOPHYSIOLOGY	SIGNS
Fresh-water	Fatigue, anxiety, difficulty breathing, fear	Water in lungs causes changes in surfactant, which in turn causes alveolar collapse.	Hypoxia, collapsed alveoli
Salt-water	Fatigue, anxiety, difficulty breathing, fear, rales, rhonchi	Hypertonic salt water pulls fluid into the alveoli.	Hypoxia, pulmonary edema

NEUROLOGICAL/ NEUROSURGICAL EMERGENCIES

Head injuries are the most common type of neurological trauma. Spinal cord trauma can also occur as a result of injuries sustained in a head injury. Head trauma most often results from motor vehicle collisions (MVCs) (Figure 37-1).

Nursing Interventions

Nursing interventions for the client with a neurological/neurosurgical emergency may include the following:

1. Monitor intracranial pressure.
2. Maintain the client in semi-Fowler's position.
3. Document vital signs hourly.
4. Assess Glasgow Coma Scale score and record hourly.
5. Administer oxygen.
6. Orient the client frequently to date and time.
7. Explain all nursing interventions.
8. Modify communication methods, such as use of a message board, depending on the client needs.

ABDOMINAL EMERGENCIES

Trauma to the upper body and torso can result in multiple abdominal injuries, from a simple contusion and bruising to a ruptured spleen.

Nursing Interventions

Nursing interventions for the client with an abdominal emergency may include the following:

1. Establish IV access with at least two large-bore catheters.
2. Monitor vital signs frequently, at least hourly.
3. Evaluate abdominal girth and bowel sounds hourly.
4. Administer antibiotics as ordered to reduce the risk of infection.
5. Monitor temperature at least every 2 hours.
6. Change saturated dressings as needed.
7. Note amount and quality of any drainage.
8. Turn client hourly from side to side.

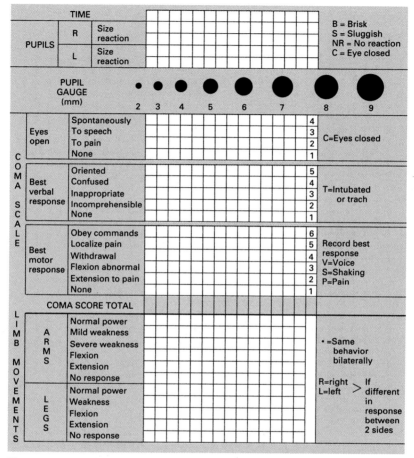

Figure 37-1 Neurological Flow Sheet, Including Glasgow Coma Scale

GENITOURINARY EMERGENCIES

Rape is defined as sexual penetration of a forceful and threatening nature with a nonconsenting person.

Straddle injuries are another type of genitourinary emergency. These injuries occur when a client falls while straddling an object, such as a fence or metal bar, thereby injuring the perineum.

Nursing Interventions

Nursing interventions for the client with genitourinary emergencies may include the following:

1. Closely monitor output.
2. Test urine for blood using dipstick.
3. Keep the client informed about all test results.
4. Maintain open and nonjudgmental communication with the client.

5. Call rape crisis center for immediate referral and assistance for the client.

6. Teach the client that the trauma does not resolve overnight and that help is available at all times.

Ocular Emergencies

Clients with objects impaled in the eye must be immediately evaluated by an ophthalmologist. An eyeball may be avulsed, or forcibly torn out of its socket, either by blunt or penetrating trauma; such an injury requires immediate referral to and treatment by an ophthalmologist. Retinal detachment is a surgical emergency, as it is one of the leading causes of accidental blindness.

Nursing Interventions

Nursing interventions for the client with an ocular emergency may include the following:

1. Maintain the client in semi-Fowler's position in cases of ocular avulsion or retinal detachment.

2. Assist the client to walk while wearing an eye patch and discuss problems that may be encountered and ways to accommodate decreased vision.

3. Instill initial eye medication and apply initial eye patch for the client.

4. Teach the client to instill eye medication.

5. Teach the client to apply eye patch.

6. Instruct the client to immediately report any visual changes or drainage.

7. Be alert and listen to the client's concerns.

MUSCULOSKELETAL EMERGENCIES

A muscle strain is the overstretching of a muscle. A sprain is defined as a twisting of the joint with partial rupture of ligaments, which can cause injury to surrounding tissue. A dislocation is the displacement of a bone from its joint. A fracture is a break in the continuity of a bone. Fat emboli from the fracture site can develop and cause severe respiratory problems if they settle in the pulmonary system.

Nursing Interventions

Nursing interventions for the client with a musculoskeletal emergency may include the following:

1. Administer pain medications as ordered.

2. Immobilize affected body part.

3. Elevate injured extremity.

4. Apply ice packs, as directed.

5. Assess the client's pulse, skin color, capillary refill, and ability to move the fingers and toes every 30 minutes.

6. Ask the client about sensation in the injured body part.

7. Apply an elastic bandage for compression in cases of a sprain.

8. Teach the client to care for the cast.

9. Teach the client exercises to minimize muscle atrophy.

10. Teach crutch walking, if needed.

SOFT-TISSUE EMERGENCIES

Minor abrasions, lacerations, puncture wounds, contusions, bites of all varieties (human, insect, animal, and snake), and burn injuries fall into this category.

Nursing Interventions

Nursing interventions for the client with a soft-tissue injury may include the following:

1. Prepare client for cleansing and possible suturing of wound.
2. Cleanse wound thoroughly with soap and water.
3. Administer tetanus intramuscularly (IM).
4. Teach the client to keep the wound and sutures dry and clean.
5. Apply a topical antibiotic and clean dressing, if indicated.
6. Teach the client to remove and change the dressing if it becomes dirty or wet.
7. Tell the client to return for additional care if wound becomes red, edematous, or painful or exhibits purulent discharge.

POISONING AND OVERDOSES

Poisoning and overdoses can be accidental or intentional. Poison control centers are the best source of antidote information for the client suffering from poisoning or overdose.

Nursing Interventions

Nursing interventions for the client with an overdose may include the following:

1. Manage the ABCs and stabilize the client.
2. Administer antidotes to toxins.
3. Document the client's response.
4. Encourage the client to share reasons for overdose.
5. Refer to help groups.
6. Assist the client in identifying different methods of coping.
7. Encourage family counseling.

ENVIRONMENTAL/ TEMPERATURE EMERGENCIES

Exposure to extremes of heat and cold can be potentially life threatening. Severe cold, or hypothermia, can occur both in very cold weather and from prolonged submersion in cold water. Heart rate and metabolic rate fall, and cardiac arrest may follow. Frostbite is another potentially dangerous result of exposure to cold (Table 37–3). Table 37–4 compares heat injuries.

Medical–Surgical Management

Medical

For those exposed to extreme cold, rewarming is essential to resuscitation. The body's core (rectal) temperature must be taken. Gradual warming must be initiated using warm blankets, warmed oxygen, warmed IV fluids, warmed nasogastric tubes, and, in extreme instances, warmed enemas. Resuscitation should continue until the body has reached a core temperature of at least 34.4°C (94°F).

For frostbite, rewarming of the exposed body part is indicated. If the frostbite is severe, rapid rewarming is

Table 37–3 DEGREES OF FROSTBITE SEVERITY

DEGREE	SYMPTOMS	TREATMENT
Mild	Skin is cold to touch, pale, tingling, and numb, with a prickly sensation	Use blankets, warm clothing to warm cold flesh
Moderate	Affects deeper body tissue; skin appears waxy and is puffy to touch and itchy and burning with pain	Use gloves, blankets, warm clothing to warm cold flesh, observe closely for deeper injuries
Severe	Blistering, damage to all layers of soft tissue; flesh appears lifeless and is hard to the touch; no pain sensation in or ability to move frozen area	Initiate emergency rewarming in an ED using warm-water baths at 40.6° C (105°F); observe carefully for increased edema

Table 37–4 COMPARISON OF HEAT INJURIES

TYPE	SYMPTOMS	TREATMENT
Heat cramps	Muscle cramps in arms, legs, and abdomen	Move client to cool, shady area. Slowly administer copious amounts of water. Reevaluate.
Heat exhaustion	Diaphoresis, with pale, moist, cool skin, headache, weakness, dizziness; muscle cramps, nausea, chills, tachypnea, confusion, tingling of hands and feet	Move client to cool, shady area. Loosen/remove constrictive clothing. Pour water over client; place client near fan. Encourage client to slowly drink water. Elevate client's legs. Reevaluate.
Heat stroke (a medical emergency)	Red, flushed, hot, dry skin; no diaphoresis	Reduce client's body temperature by removing client's clothing and pouring cool water over client. Start two large-bore IV lines. Use fan to cool client. Place client on cardiac monitor. Elevate client's legs. Assess client's vital signs, especially core (rectal) temperature. Check for neurological signs (confused, combative, disoriented). Check client's core (rectal) temperature frequently.

Developed from U.S. Army Training Support Command Protocols.

essential. This involves placing the frozen area in warm-water baths not exceeding 40.6°C (105°F). Tetanus should be administered. Acute pain should be treated with analgesics.

For heat injuries, rapidly reducing the body's temperature is vital. Supplemental oxygen may be administered. Pouring cool water over the client, chilling IV fluids, and fanning the client will accelerate the cooling process.

Nursing Interventions

Nursing interventions for the client with a temperature/environmental injury may include the following:

Hypothermia
1. Administer supplemental oxygen.
2. Monitor cardiac response carefully.
3. If CPR is in progress, continue until the client's core temperature reaches 94° F and cardiac status is evaluated.
4. Administer warmed IV fluids.
5. Place warmed blankets on the client.

Hyperthermia
1. Remove the client's clothing.
2. Pour cool water over the client.
3. Use large fan to cool the client.
4. Administer chilled IV fluids.
5. Administer supplemental oxygen.

6. Initiate cardiac monitoring.
7. Evaluate client's neurological status with reference to orientation to time, person, and place.
8. Measure core temperature every 30 minutes to assess progress.

MULTIPLE-SYSTEM TRAUMA

Multiple-system trauma is injury sustained in more than one body system.

Nursing Interventions

Nursing interventions for the client with multiple-system trauma may include the following:

1. Maintain open airway.
2. Initiate rescue breathing.
3. Assist with insertion of endotracheal tube.
4. Maintain pulse oximetry reading at 94% to 99%.
5. Start multiple large-bore IV lines.
6. Explain all nursing/medical interventions to client.
7. Provide emotional and physiological support to client and family as much as possible throughout resuscitation.

APPENDIX A
ABBREVIATIONS

ʒ	dram
℥	ounce
♏	minum
ā	before
ABC	airway, breathing, circulation
ABG	arterial blood gases
a.c.	before meals
AD	right ear
ad lib	freely, as desired
ADL	activities of daily living
AEB	as evidenced by
AP	anterior/posterior
AP	apical pulse
AS	left ear
bid	twice a day
BMR	basal metabolic rate
B&O	belladonna and opium
BP	blood pressure
c	cup
C	Celsius
c̄	with
CABG	coronary artery bypass graft
CaCl₂	calcium chloride
C & S	culture and sensitivity
CBC	complete blood count
cc	cubic centimeter
CF	cystic fibrosis
CFTR	cystic fibrosis transmembrane regulator
CHF	congestive heart failure
cm	centimeter
CMS	circulation, movement, sensation
CNS	central nervous system
CO₂	carbon dioxide
COLD	chronic obstructive lung disease
COPD	chronic obstructive pulmonary disease
CPR	cardiopulmonary resuscitation
CSF	cerebrospinal fluid
D₅W	dextrose 5% in water
dc	discontinue
DKA	diabetic ketoacidosis
dL	deciliter
DNR	do not resuscitate
dr	dram, or ʒ
DRG	diagnosis-related group
DVT	deep vein thrombosis
ECF	extracellular fluid
ECG (EKG)	electrocardiogram
ED	emergency department
EEG	electroencephalograph
EENT	eyes, ears, nose, and throat

ESR	erythrocyte sedimentation rate
ESRD	end-stage renal disease
ET	endotracheal
ETT	endotracheal tube
FBD	fibrocystic breast disease
FBS	fasting blood sugar
fl	fluid
FOBT	fecal occult blood test
g	gram
GCS	Glasgow Coma Scale
GERD	gastrointestinal reflux disease
GFR	glomerular filtration rate
GI	gastrointestinal
gr	grain
gtt	drop
GTT	glucose tolerance test
gtt/min	drops per minute
GU	genitourinary
h	hour(s)
H₂O	water
HBₛAG	hepatitis B surface antigen
H&H	hemoglobin and hematocrit
HCl	hydrochloric acid
Hct	hematocrit
HDL	high density lipoprotein
Hep B	hepatitis B
Hgb	hemoglobin
HHNK	hyperosmolar hyperglycemic nonketotic syndrome
HIV	human immunodeficiency virus
h.s.	hour of sleep
HTN	hypertension
IABP	intra-aortic balloon pump
IADL	instrumental activities of daily living
I&O	intake and output
ICF	intracellular fluid
ID	intradermal
IGT	impaired glucose tolerance
IM	intramuscular
INR	International Normalized Ratio
IOL	intraocular lens
IOP	intraocular pressure
IV	intravenous
IVP	intravenous push, intravenous pyelogram
IVPB	intravenous piggyback
KCl	potassium chloride
kg	kilogram
KUB	kidneys/ureters/bladder
KVO	keep vein open
L	liter
LDL	low density lipoprotein

LES	lower esophageal sphincter	**PT**	prothrombin time
LLQ	left lower quadrant	**PTT**	partial thromboplastin time
LMP	last menstrual period	**q**	*quaque,* Latin for "every"
LOC	level of consciousness	**qd**	every day
LP	lumbar puncture	**qh**	very hour
LUQ	left upper quadrant	**qid**	four times a day
MAR	medication administration record	**qod**	every other day
		qs	quantity sufficient
mcg	microgram	**q2h**	every 2 hours
(or μg)		**RBC**	red blood count, red blood cell
mEq	milliequivalent		
mEq/L	milliequivalents per liter	**RDS**	respiratory distress syndrome
mg	milligram		
MgCl	magnesium chloride	**RICE**	rest, ice, compression, elevation
MgSO$_4$	magnesium sulfate		
MI	myocardial infarction	**RLQ**	right lower quadrant
min	minute	**ROM**	range of motion
mL	milliliter	**R/T**	related to
mm^3	cubic millimeter	**RTI**	respiratory tract infection
mm Hg	millimeters of mercury	**RUQ**	right upper quadrant
mOsm/	milliosmoles/kilogram	**s̄**	without
kg		**SaO$_2$**	oxygen saturation
MS	morphine sulfate	**SC/SQ**	subcutaneous
NaCl	sodium chloride	**SL**	sublingual
NG	nasogastric	**STAT**	*statim,* Latin for "immediately"
NIC	Nursing Interventions Classification		
		supp	suppository
NOC	Nursing Outcomes Classification	**susp**	suspension
NPO	*nil per os,* Latin for "nothing by mouth"	**tab**	tablet
		TENS	transcutaneous electrical nerve stimulation
O$_2$	oxygen		
O&P	ova and parasite	**T$_4$**	thyroxine
OD	right eye	**t.i.d.**	three times a day
OS	left eye	**TPN**	total parenteral nutrition
OTC	over-the-counter	**TPR**	temperature, pulse, respirations
OU	both eyes		
p̄	after	**Tr or**	tincture
Pap	Papanicolaou test	**tinct**	
PCA	patient-controlled analgesia	**TSE**	testicular self-examination
PCO$_2$	partial pressure of carbon	**T$_3$**	triiodothyronine
(PaCO$_2$)	dioxide	**U**	unit
PERRLA	pupils equal, round, reactive to light and accommodation	**UA**	routine urinalysis
		URQ	upper right quadrant
pH	potential hydrogen	**VDRL**	venereal disease research laboratory
po	*per os,* Latin for "by mouth"		
PO$_2$	partial pressure of oxygen	**VLDL**	very low-density lipoprotein
(PaO$_2$)			
PPBS	post prandial blood sugar	**VMA**	vanillylmandelic acid
(PPG)	(glucose)	**VS**	vital signs
PRN	*pro re nata,* Latin for "as required"	**WBC**	white blood cell, white blood count
PROM	passive range of motion	**WNL**	within normal limits

APPENDIX B
NANDA NURSING
DIAGNOSES 2001-2002

Activity Intolerance
Risk for Activity Intolerance
Impaired Adjustment
Ineffective Airway Clearance
Latex Allergy Response
Risk for Latex Allergy Response
Anxiety
Death Anxiety
Risk for Aspiration
Risk for Impaired Parent/Infant/Child Attachment
Autonomic Dysreflexia
Disturbed Body Image
Risk for Imbalanced Body Temperature
Bowel Incontinence
Effective Breastfeeding
Ineffective Breastfeeding
Interrupted Breastfeeding
Ineffective Breathing Pattern
Decreased Cardiac Output
Caregiver Role Strain
Risk for Caregiver Role Strain
Impaired Verbal Communication
Decisional Conflict (Specify)
Parenteral Role Conflict
Acute Confusion
Chronic Confusion
Constipation
Perceived Constipation
Risk for Constipation
Ineffective Coping
Ineffective Community Coping
Readiness for Enhanced Community Coping
Defensive Coping
Compromised Family Coping
Disabled Family Coping
Readiness for Enhanced Family Coping
Ineffective Denial
Impaired Dentition
Risk for Delayed Development
Diarrhea
Risk for Disuse Syndrome
Deficient Diversional Activities
Disturbed Energy Field
Impaired Environmental Interpretation Syndrome
Adult Failure to Thrive
Risk for Falls

Dysfunctional Family Processes: Alcoholism
Interrupted Family Processes
Fatigue
Fear
Deficient Fluid Volume
Excess Fluid Volume
Risk for Deficient Fluid Volume
Risk for Imbalanced Fluid Volume
Impaired Gas Exchange
Anticipatory Grieving
Dysfunctional Grieving
Delayed Growth and Development
Risk for Disproportionate Growth
Ineffective Health Maintenance
Health-Seeking Behaviors (Specify)
Impaired Home Maintenance
Hopelessness
Hyperthermia
Hypothermia
Disturbed Personal Identity
Functional Urinary Incontinence
Reflex Urinary Incontinence
Stress Urinary Incontinence
Total Urinary Incontinence
Urge Urinary Incontinence
Risk for Urge Urinary Incontinence
Disorganized Infant Behavior
Risk for Disorganized Infant Behavior
Readiness for Enhanced Organized Infant Behavior
Ineffective Infant Feeding Pattern
Risk for Infection
Risk for Injury
Risk for Perioperative-Positioning Injury
Decreased Intracranial Adaptive Capacity
Deficient Knowledge
Risk for Loneliness
Impaired Memory
Impaired Bed Mobility
Impaired Physical Mobility
Impaired Wheelchair Mobility
Nausea
Unilateral Neglect
Noncompliance

Imbalanced **N**utrition: Less than Body Requirements

Imbalanced **N**utrition: More than Body Requirements

Risk for Imbalanced **N**utrition: More than Body Requirements

Impaired **O**ral Mucous Membrane

Acute **P**ain

Chronic **P**ain

Impaired **P**arenting

Risk for Impaired **P**arenting

Risk for **P**eripheral Neurovascular Dysfunction

Risk for **P**oisoning

Post-Trauma Syndrome

Risk for **P**ost-Trauma Syndrome

Powerlessness

Risk for **P**owerlessness

Ineffective **P**rotection

Rape-Trauma Syndrome

Rape-Trauma Syndrome: Compound Reaction

Rape-Trauma Syndrome: Silent Reaction

Relocation Stress Syndrome

Risk for **R**elocation Stress Syndrome

Ineffective **R**ole Performance

Bathing/Hygiene **S**elf-Care Deficit

Dressing/Grooming **S**elf-Care Deficit

Feeding **S**elf-Care Deficit

Toileting **S**elf-Care Deficit

Chronic Low **S**elf-Esteem

Situational Low **S**elf-Esteem

Risk for Situational Low **S**elf-Esteem

Self-Mutilation

Risk for **S**elf-Mutilation

Disturbed **S**ensory Perception (Specify: Visual, Auditory, Kinesthetic, Gustatory, Tactile, Olfactory)

Sexual Dysfunction

Ineffective **S**exuality Patterns

Impaired **S**kin Integrity

Risk for Impaired **S**kin Integrity

Sleep Deprivation

Disturbed **S**leep Pattern

Impaired **S**ocial Interaction

Social Isolation

Chronic **S**orrow

Spiritual Distress

Risk for **S**piritual Distress

Readiness for Enhanced **S**piritual Well-Being

Risk for **S**uffocation

Risk for **S**uicide

Delayed **S**urgical Recovery

Impaired **S**wallowing

Effective **T**herapeutic Regimen Management

Ineffective **T**herapeutic Regimen Management

Ineffective Community **T**herapeutic Regimen Management

Ineffective Family **T**herapeutic Regimen Management

Ineffective **T**hermoregulation

Disturbed **T**hought Processes

Impaired **T**issue Integrity

Ineffective **T**issue Perfusion (Specify Type: Renal, Cerebral, Cardio-pulmonary, Gastrointestinal, Peripheral)

Impaired **T**ransfer Ability

Risk for **T**rauma

Impaired **U**rinary Elimination

Urinary Retention

Impaired Spontaneous **V**entilation

Dysfunctional **V**entilatory Weaning Response

Risk for Other-Directed **V**iolence

Risk for Self-Directed **V**iolence

Impaired **W**alking

Wandering

INDEX